Magic Search Words

HEALTH

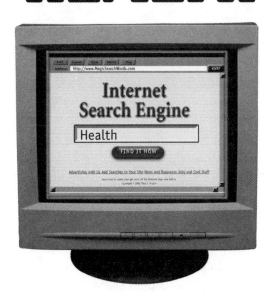

Internet
Search Engine

Health

FIND IT NOW

Advertising with Us Add Searches to Your Site News and Resources Jobs and Cool Stuff

Learn how to create your get more of the Internet than ever before.
Copyright © 2002 Paul J. Bright

The Magic Search Word Series

Scholarships
Jobs
Health
Homework
Business
Law
Personal Finance
Animal and Pet Care
Environment

Free! Access to www.MagicSearchWords.com

Each of the Magic Search Words books provides you with free access to the custom programmed Magic Search Words web site.

MagicSearchWords.com automates the creation of search strings, so that creating search strings and submitting them to the best search engines is even faster and easier than ever.

You may go to www.MagicSearchWords.com anytime once you have purchased or downloaded a book.

Thank you for your interest in improving your life!

Magic Search Words

HEALTH

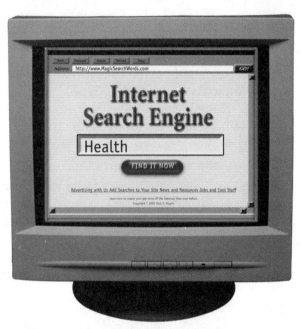

Strategies and Search Tactics to Discover the Best of the Internet

Paul J. Krupin

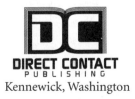

DIRECT CONTACT
PUBLISHING
Kennewick, Washington

Books are available in quantity for promotional or premium use.
Write to the Director of Special Sales,
Direct Contact Publishing,
P. O. Box 6726, Kennewick, WA 99336,
Email info@MagicSearchWords.com
or call (509) 545–2707.

www.MagicSearchWords.com

ISBN 1–885035–11–X (softcover)
ISBN 1–885035–15–2 (e-book)

Cover and Interior Design & Typesetting by Desktop Miracles, Inc., Stowe, VT

Library of Congress Cataloging-in-Publication Data

Krupin, Paul J.
    Magic search words: health—strategies and tactics to discover the best of the Internet / Paul J. Krupin
        p.   cm.
    ISBN 1–885035–11–X (softcover)
    ISBN 1–885035–15–2 (e-book)
    1. Medicine, Popular—Computer network resources.   2. Health care (Medical)—Computer networks.   3. Internet (Computer network).
I. Title.   II. Series.
025.06'65—dc21

Printed in the United States of America
07 06 05 04 03 02   10 9 8 7 6 5 4 3 2 1

To all the children,
For they shall inherit our knowledge,
hopes, dreams and visions.

Disclaimer

Even a book like this has limitations. This book was written to provide information on the subject of searching and finding information on the Internet. It is sold with the understanding that the publisher and author are not engaged in rendering legal, accounting or other professional services. If expert assistance is required, then the services of a competent professional should be sought.

It is not the intent of this book to cover all the information that is available on this topic from other experts and creative people who also write on this subject. Rather it is intended to complement, amplify, and supplement other available works.

Seeking medical information and valid, personal advice or guidance on the Internet is not a guaranteed endeavor. Anyone who decides this book is for them must expect to invest a lot of time and effort without any guarantee of success. Answers to your questions do not appear magically. What you read may not be totally true or relevant to your particular situation. To receive valid bona fide medical advice, you must go to a licensed certified medical practitioner.

Every effort has been made to make this book complete and as accurate as possible. However, there may be mistakes both typographical and in content. Therefore, this book should only be used as a general guide and not as the ultimate source for information on medical information online. Furthermore, this book only contains information that is current as of the printing date.

The purpose of this manual is to educate and entertain. The author and publisher shall have neither liability nor responsibility to any person or entity with respect to any loss or damage caused or alleged to be caused directly or indirectly by the information contained in this book.

If you do not wish to be bound by the above you may return this book to the publisher for a full refund.

If you love to find mistakes, please send in your corrections for the next edition.

Magic Ingredients

Foreword   xi
Preface   xiii
Acknowledgments   xv

CHAPTER 1: **INTRODUCTION**   1
- Overview
- Purpose
- Getting Started
- How To Use This Book

CHAPTER 2: **ALL ABOUT SEARCH ENGINES**   7
- True Search Engines
- Web Directories
- Virtual Libraries
- Meta-Search Engines
- The Invisible Web
- Search Engine Resources

CHAPTER 3: **MAGIC SEARCH WORDS**   15
- The Search String Technique
  - Simple Searches
  - Advanced Searches
  - Concept and Phrase Searches

CHAPTER 4: **THE MAGIC SEARCH WORDS KINGDOM**   39
- Overview of the Kingdom
- Magic Potions: The Key Search String Word Groups
- Inside the Key Medical Search String Word Groups

CHAPTER 5:   **DISCOVERING THE FOUNTAIN OF ETERNAL YOUTH**   61
- Specific Medical & Health Topics

  - Aging, Elder Care, Long-Term Care and Rehabilitation
  - Allergies, Asthma, & Immunology
  - Alternative Health & Medical Treatment
  - Blood, Circulatory & Lymphatic System
  - Bones, muscles, joints, orthopedics & physical therapy
  - Cancer
  - Chiropractic Care
  - Colds and the Flu
  - Death & Dying
  - Dental and Oral Care
  - Diabetes, Hormonal & other Immune System Disorders
  - Digestive System & Gastrointestinal Illness
  - Ears and Hearing
  - Eating, Foods and Nutrition
  - Emergencies, Poison Control & Safety
  - Eye Care & Vision
  - Family & Parenting
  - Fitness & Exercise
  - Foot Care
  - Heart Disease and Cardiology
  - Headache and Migraine
  - Infections
  - Lungs & Airways
  - Medication & Drugs
  - Men's Health
  - Mental Health & Psychiatry
  - Nervous System and Neurology
  - Physical & Developmental Disabilities
  - Plastic Surgery
  - Sex & Fertility
  - Sexual Disorders
  - Skin Care and Skin Diseases
  - Sleep Disorders
  - Social Problems, Physical, Sexual Problems
  - Sports Medicine and Injuries
  - Substance Abuse
  - Surgery
  - Tests, Tools and Calculators
  - Travel and Health
  - Women's Health
  - X-rays, Radiology and Nuclear Medicine

CHAPTER 6:   THE CASTLES OF THE KINGDOM   119
- Going from Ideas to Action
- Special Topics In Medical Health Care
- Doctors & Health Care Professionals
- Hospitals and Health Care Facilities
- Insurance & Health Care Providers
- Medical Education
- Government Agencies
- Companies & Corporations
- Professional Associations and Organizations
- Educational Institutions
- Media
- Legal Questions, Fraud or Abuse
- Free Stuff

CHAPTER 7:   CONCLUSION   137
- Avoiding Disaster
- Parting Words

APPENDIX: SUMMARY OF THE BEST HEALTH
             MAGIC SEARCH WORDS   141

Index   143

Who is Paul J. Krupin?   147

Foreword

by Meryl K. Evans

The Internet and especially its search engines have helped me tremendously in my career as a writer. Without search engines, I would have to spend hours manually tracking down needed information for interviews, articles, reviews, and other writing projects.

Whenever I needed to do research for school, I had to do it the old-fashioned way since it was pre-Internet times. That meant going to the library, organizations, and bookstores to comb for information.

That was barely a decade ago. Phenomenal changes have taken place in the world since I was a student trying to collect the right information to get a good grade. When I entered college, computers weren't quite on every desk. Four years later when I entered the work force, fellow co-workers and I had our own computers.

Just because the search engines and other Internet resources are there for the taking, information won't come to you without your help. Libraries and references still require the crucial and critical skills of knowing how to ask the right questions to search and find the answers.

With search engines having indexed billions of Web pages, it's become a game of looking for a needle in the haystack. We have to give it a hand so it can return the favor of finding what we need without providing irrelevant and overwhelming results.

Online searching is becoming a necessary skill that is in demand for people in all walks of life. It's for the student who is trying to get a good grade on a thesis. It's for the parent who is trying to handle a parenting issue. It's for the professional who is trying to advance in a career. It's for the traveler who is looking for that next exciting destination.

The *Magic Search Words* series provides you with the basic building blocks that expert searchers use. Not only will it give you strategies to support you in your current search efforts, but also it will empower you to learn more and benefit from search engines to help you in other areas of your life.

The book is an incredibly fast read and it'll show you how to conduct effective searches. With a little practice and advice, online searching will become a habit and open new worlds for you.

MERYL K. EVANS
AUTHOR
WWW.MERYL.NET
PLANO, TEXAS

Preface

This book is all about Internet wizardry.

This is not just about technology, but rather the focus is on *YOU*, the person who sits at the computer.

This book teaches *YOU* how to select the right string of words for your search. The words you select and enter are the *Magic Search Words.*

It's a remarkable book really; the search string technique described here empowers you to get more valuable, relevant, and immediately useful information off the Internet than any other search engine tool ever created.

Search strings are a breakthrough in getting the best and most relevant information as quick as a click. They work and they can help you get results.

You will do best if you know what you want and learn the technical language of your chosen area of interest.

If you don't yet know what you want, that's OK. You'll have plenty of opportunity to find out and there are plenty of things to look at and experience. Eventually, after learning how to search, you'll want to step back and take a breather.

Use this time wisely. Plan your approach and prepare your tools. Have your off line letters, applications, letters of recommendation and references available and ready to be adapted for your use.

Then follow the steps: Search, Find, Match and Apply. These simple strategies, tactics and magic words will cut through the clutter and get you right to what you need and want the most.

Most people read through this book quickly one time. Then they go back and read it again, doing the recommended searches, to gain solid experience and knowledge. Then, you can begin to fly.

Acknowledgments

I wish to acknowledge with the deepest possible respect and thanks my parents, Helene and Murray Krupin, who gave me the most profound gift anyone can ever receive, the love of learning. My grandmother, Ida Sokol, still serves as a stalwart rock of strength and inspiration, her business sense, spiritual devotion, and dedication to finding satisfaction in service to others has shaped my own destiny into a satisfying life of public service. Working next to you as a child and a teenager Aunt Cookie, you taught me the first magic words "Can I help you". Aunt Judy, thank you for being a first class librarian and a critical reviewer with a superb eye for detail. Uncle Jack and Aunt Priscilla, thanks for sitting me down, helping me in time of need, and telling me in no uncertain terms that I have a duty to get back to business. To my family, your love, counsel, words, thoughts and feelings, conveyed to me throughout my youth, allowed the sparks of creativity to grow into a firestorm, and have helped me dedicate, channel and focus my energy towards the creation of tools that can be used to better humankind.

To my numerous colleagues in government and industry, I recognize your talents and skills and it is with great pleasure I now seek to share some of the energy, expertise, and talent you have imparted to me. Being around you and watching you work in managing the government has been a galvanizing and adventurous experience. Watching you tackle the problems of society with the tools and technologies available to us has infected me with a sense of responsibility for humanity. Thank you for allowing me to be a contributor. Your mentoring has helped motivate and shape the creation of the tools contained in these books.

Ben Kaplan, I want to say thank you for identifying the need for this book. Your own efforts, writings, enthusiasm and success motivated me to strive to create these tactics and once the ideas were conceived, to follow your lead and share them with others so they may benefit.

Dan Poynter, self publishing guru and mentor extraordinaire, you once again have shaped the world by inspiring creativity and helping a self-published author through the gauntlet to publishing success. Thank you!

Barry Kerrigan and Del LeMond, you guys are capable of much more than just Desktop Miracles, you are true alchemists, magicians of the printed word and graphic arts. I also want to thank computer wiz Tony Dolman, of Networks Northwest for keeping my computers humming and recognize the extraordinary talents and programming skills of Don Short of One World Telecommunications, without whom none of this would be possible. To Kathleen Stidham, thank you for your timely review and insights.

To agent Jeff Herman, thank you for trying! To the dozen or so east coast publishers who rejected the first version of this book, thank you! If you hadn't rejected the original manuscripts, the techniques and tactics contained in the present version of the *Magic Search Words* series would not have been created.

To my editors, Judith Whitehead, the mystery editor in New York, Angela K. Durden, and Meryl K. Evans, thank you for your hurricane force creativity and talents. Yes, I am a once-upon-a-time lawyer who still types with two fingers, thankfully knows when to ask for help, and hopefully knows how to graciously receive it. You have tactfully and elegantly guided me through the collaborative process and helped me create this incredible tool for educating and helping people with simplicity, brevity and style. Your comments and insights have helped redefine and reinvent the concepts in this book series again and again. Here's to many more happy revisions!

Most important of all, to my wife Nancy, and my two dynamite daughters, you provide me with support and inspire me to achieve. May I continue to make you proud.

PAUL KRUPIN
KENNEWICK, WASHINGTON 2002

one

Introduction

Overview

The Magic Search Word books present you with an entirely new set of easy-to-learn Internet search skills and techniques. You can use these to increase your knowledge, skills, financial success, health, and the overall quality of your life, as well as those around you.

These powerful books are written with a user view at their core. They show you exactly how to search the Internet and find the best life-saving health and medical information available quicker, faster and easier than you ever imagined possible.

You will be amazed, even if you think you know everything there is to know about the Internet. You are about to learn that there is a whole new universe at your fingertips. So be open and get ready to learn some very simple, yet mind-boggling, powerful techniques.

These books teach you how to use magic search words, create "search strings", and use special techniques like the search word rotation, the minus .com trick, searching with phrases or concepts, with personal, social of family information, or by subject, sources, date, location and much, much more.

These methods were developed by carefully distilling trial and error experience, analyzing the results from thousands and thousands of individual searches and by seeking ways to leverage the ever-improving Intenet and search engine technologies.

They have been reviewed and endorsed by experts in the field of library science as well as by subject matter experts in the various topics addressed by each book.

And they deliver. You can find what you want. As quick as a click!

We encourage you to read these books carefully and then get on line and search. Use Magic Search Word techniques frequently so that you fully benefit from the powerful knowledge contained on the Internet.

We hope that you will use what you learn so that *you* may profit personally. Then, please share your newly found knowledge, skills, capability and experience with others so that they might profit as well.

Purpose

This book is all about searching the Internet for health and medical information. You can quickly find the really valuable and useful, even life-saving information, on the Internet if you learn how to do three things:

1. how to use search engines;
2. how to select the right search words; and
3. how to string the words together to do an effective search.

The key to being successful is using what I call Internet "search strings."

A search string is simply a series or *a string of key words* that you enter into the search engine to find what you are looking for. It can be two words, four words, six words or even ten or eleven words in a row.

Once you learn how to create search strings, there is no bit of information that you can't find.

To understand the power of the string search, you have to understand the paradox of the Internet. The amount of really incredible information of real value on the Internet has exploded.

From 1998 to 2001 government agencies, universities, professional organizations, and companies went online in a really big way. They keep putting more, better, and higher quality information online every day.

While the information available was exploding, the search engines were also getting easier to use. Technology has made it quicker and easier to reach out and grab that information. Every day brings new advances. Computers are faster, plus Internet connections are better than ever and continue getting better every day.

But guess what? The technology is changing so fast that most people haven't yet come to grips yet with the human factors involved in taking advantage of these newly developed powers.

So much has changed that no one really knows what's out there any more. There is so much information floating out there in cyberspace, yet no one seems to know how to find the good stuff—the real gold—*information*. Information is power. It is an unfortunate paradox; we're all dressed up, we know where we want to go, but we have no idea on how to get there!

Enter "Magic Search Words" and the "Search String Technique". These methods are simple and easy-to-learn methods that you can use to improve what you get off the Internet.

Magic search words and the string search technique will enable you to tap into the power of the Internet like never before.

These techniques can be applied to searching anything. Once you learn how to use magic search words and create your own search strings, you will be able to search for information and find new opportunities easier than you ever imagined possible. It will become a tool that you incorporate into your every day pursuits for the rest of your life.

And best of all—it won't be hard to learn at all. Are you ready? Let's get started.

Getting Started

You are searching the Internet, so you will obviously need a computer with access to the Internet, a printer, and the fastest Internet connection you can find. The faster the service, the less time you have to sit and stare at the computer screen while your searches are executed.

Software is also important. You will need to be able to browse or surf the Internet using the best available software you can find. The browsing software should have come on your computer, whether you use a PC or Mac, or you can get the browser and periodic updates when you sign up for Internet access.

To make sure that you have the newest browser available, download the updates directly from the Internet. The two biggest names out there right now are Microsoft Internet Explorer and Netscape Navigator with Opera and Mozilla gaining on them. You can download these for free.

Your computer is ground zero. The most important thing to do here is learn how to use your software and use it efficiently. Part of this is trial and error, but some of it is as simple as finding the "help" button and reading the frequently asked questions (FAQ's) or other helpful information that is invariably tucked away in there.

What you will want to do with the browser that you are using is create a series of bookmarks or favorite folders, and a series of sub-folders or directories.

Once you have determined what search engine you like the best, you can:

- set the browser window to default to your favorite search engine whenever you start up your Internet browser; or
- create a shortcut to your favorite search engine and place it on your desktop so that you can open your favorite search engine with one click.

How to Use This Book

In this book, you will be learning how to conduct your own custom searches. To help you learn and master the techniques, you will conduct numerous searches one at a time.

*We will tell you what words to enter by underlining the
actual search words to enter on your computer screen like this:*

Search engines

All you have to do go to your favorite search engine, enter the words and click.

My favorite true search engine is Google. You can get to it by opening up your Internet browser and by entering the words

www.google.com

Try it. You can, of course, use your favorite search engine or any of the other types of search engines, directories or databases that strike your fancy.

You will get to use many of these other types of search engines as you learn more about searching using this book.

Most people read through this book quickly one time. Then they go back and read it again, doing many of the recommended searches, to gain solid searching experience and knowledge.

Then, they do a self-assessment, making lists of the areas that interest and apply specifically to them. Take some time to get familiar with health information in general, and learn about how to create great search strings.

Then, you will be ready to embark on a systematic search to identify and apply for the opportunities you discover. If you learn the techniques and implement them faithfully, you will be successful.

Free! Access to www.MagicSearchWords.com

Each of the Magic Search Words books provides you with free access to the custom programmed Magic Search Words web site.

MagicSearchWords.com automates the creation of search strings, so that creating search strings and submitting them to the best search engines is even faster and easier than ever.

You may go to www.MagicSearchWords.com anytime once you have purchased or downloaded a book.

Thank you for your interest in improving your life!

QUICKSTART

Go to www.Google.com.

CREATE A SEARCH STRING

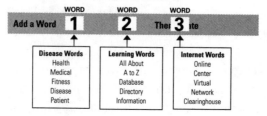

Disease Words	Learning Words	Internet Words
Health	All About	Online
Medical	A to Z	Center
Fitness	Database	Virtual
Disease	Directory	Network
Patient	Information	Clearinghouse

Select one word from each column and create a search string like this:

Health A to Z Online

Then search on the words you selected. Study the results. Surf through the web sites you find and learn what they have to offer. Enjoy what you find.

Then create another search string using different words and search again.

two

All About Search Engines

There are several different types of search engines on the Internet. You will search better if you learn about them and how they work.

True Search Engines

A search engine is a Web site that is home to a specialized software program that helps you find relevant information.

"True" search engines do not search the Internet every time you enter a search term. The search engine program visits Web sites all over the Internet every so often, say once a month, and creates what is called an "index," a big vast snapshot of the pages it has visited.

When you enter a search word, the program then searches out all references to that search word in the index of the web sites it has visited. If it finds the search word, it brings back the Web site address, the universal resource locator, or URL for short.

True search engines include Google.com, Infoseek.com, Hotbot.com, and AltaVista.com. Each of these big automated search engines has four basic parts:

1. A "robot" or "spider" of some sort that automatically collects links, titles, and text from Internet sites at a certain frequency established by the people who own and manage the engine.

   What this means is that each search engine is using its own specific set of criteria to decide what kinds of information to include in its database (*see* below), so each search engine you use can bring back different kinds of information, even when you use the exact same search terms.

2. A database where the collected information is stored and maintained. All the information that the spiders or robots bring back is dumped into a database from which your queries will be drawn. The more frequently the spiders are sent out, the fresher the information in the database will be.

3. An index where the collected information is cataloged for queries and retrieval. The people who own and manage the engine also establish the index. So, when you enter search terms the search engine will give you results that are listed according to the particular engine's own ranking system. Using the same search terms, each search engine can bring up a slightly different list of results because each uses a different set of criteria to determine the ranking or relevance of sites.

4. A search tool that allows the user to ask the database index for relevant sites.

Thus, when you do a search at a search engine, you actually do not search the Web, but rather you query the search engine's index of the Web. Using its index saves you time and makes the search process manageable.

All indexes collect large numbers of links, and this is both a benefit and a problem.

On the plus side, a large number of Web sites will be identified when you do a search. This will give you a complete set of data on what is out there on the Internet.

On the down side, it is very difficult to read through all the Web sites returned, and many, many of them will have little or no true relevance to your search.

True Search Engines:

> All the Web
> Alta Vista
> Excite
> Go
> Google
> Hotbot
> Iwon
> Lycos
> Magellan
> Teoma
> Vivisimo (clustering tool)
> WebCrawler

Web Directories

A Web directory is completely different than a true search engine. It is an Internet site that contains information that have been examined and categorized in a directory.

A machine creates some directory sites, while one or more human beings create the vast majority.

Instead of sending out spiders, a Web directory uses people to review and index sites using a rigid set of criteria for deciding what sites to include and exclude from the directory. These people not only look at content, but also at the quality of the site and the user experience. This is a manpower and time-consuming process and means that a Web directory will contain fewer sites than a search engine, although the sites and links are, arguably, of a better quality.

Another distinguishing feature is that a typical directory site allows you to browse through a tree of categories, sub-categories, sub-sub-categories, etc. With a search engine, you need to actually search, using either individual terms or search strings; you cannot simply click around.

Directories allow you to do just that—find things by clicking around and seeing what there is to see.

Yahoo, Netscape, and MSN are directories. Yahoo, Magellan, and Galaxy are large collections of categorized Internet sites and documents organized according to some intelligent and easy to navigate scheme.

About.com is a directory maintained by experts, called editors. About.com competitively hires over 700 expert editors, each of whom maintains the quality and content of each section of this directory.

Directories:

> About.com
> Britannica
> LookSmart
> NBCi (formerly SNAP)
> Netscape
> Microsoft Network (MSN)
> Open Directory
> Yahoo

Virtual Libraries

Numerous government agencies and universities house highly technical computerized catalog systems that are extremely large called *Virtual Libraries*. The Library of Congress hosts one of the largest in the United States. Originally, CERN created the 3W Virtual Library, in Switzerland, but it is now maintained by a consortium of institutions, including MIT.

If you search on the words "virtual libraries" you find a huge number of specialized cataloging systems for everything from microbiology to legal documents.

Meta-Search Engines

These are highly user-friendly Web sites that allow you to simultaneously send a single query to multiple search engines, directories, or specialized databases.

The Meta-Search Engine will then retrieve, combine, organize, and evaluate the results, often eliminating the duplicates, and ranking the reliability of the combined results. Some bring back all the results in one list; some let you see each source search engines results individually.

Meta-search Engines (or Multi-search Engines)

Ask Jeeves
Cyber 411
Chubba
Dogpile
Inference Fund
Mamma
MetaCrawler
MetaFind
One2Seek
Savvy Search (Savvy)

The Invisible Web

Nowadays specialized search engines, virtual libraries, and databases are all over the Web. Search engine programming and software has become readily available, and people use these technologies to entice people to visit their Web sites for the valuable information that is kept there.

Specialized search databases are often not indexed by search engine spiders. This is called the *invisible Web.*

How do you access this invisible information? Do a search!

Create your search string using the key, magic words:

invisible Web
invisible Web tutorial

Do these searches one at a time. Read the results on the Web pages that strike your fancy.

Learn about the incredible and vast amount of valuable information that is hidden from the search engines.

The invisible web resources are of crucial importance when you are looking for high quality medical, health and pharmaceutical data and information.

Most of the most current and accurate information on diseases and medications maintained by government agencies, professional associations, and medical service and pharmaceutical companies or organizations are housed in searchable online databases.

You find these by searching for these specialized web resources using the key magic search "learning words" and "Internet Words".

Search Engine Resources

One of the easiest ways to find out what search engines, directories, and software are out there is to go to a major engine you recognize or like, type in the words "search engines" and see what results are listed.

There are many sites that will explain all these searching tools in detail, list links, and point you in the right direction if you are looking for something in particular.

For quick reference, here is a summary list of some of the most powerful search strings you can use to get current and accurate information about search engines and the most popular sites:

search engines
search engine watch
search engine showdown
search engine comparison chart

Do these searches and learn as much as you want about search engines. You will learn that there are several types of search engines to choose from:

Major search engines include the most popular or important services from all over the world. They are generally commercial sites that are very well-maintained, and many will contain both search engines and directories you can browse.

Paid listings search engines where listings are bought and sold (*e.g.,* companies pay to be high on the return search list).

Reward search engines offer cash, prizes, or other goodies to those who use them.

News search engines search for the latest news stories from carefully selected media information sources on the Web. These services can provide exceptionally good results for current event searching because they will spider only the news sites once or twice a day. Thus, the results are unusually focused and up-to-date.

Specialty search engines are available to help you find more than just Web pages and Web sites. Here are search engines that will search through specialized search engines, newsgroups, directories, specialized search databases, mailing lists, software catalogs, and more.

Kids search engines are usually more like "safe havens," directories maintained by people who carefully select sites to serve the beneficial interests of children. They cover things that kids really enjoy and they carefully exclude sites that parents and teachers might find inappropriate for kids, such as those that deal with explicit sexual matters, pornography, violence, hate speech, gambling, and drug use.

Metacrawlers allow searches to be sent to several search engines all at once. The results are then combined and returned on one or more pages for convenient viewing, with duplicates eliminated, ranked in order of importance, or by relevance, with regard to your search string.

Desktop search utilities are software programs that let you search the Internet from your desktop.

QUICKSTART
Go to www.Google.com.

CREATE A SEARCH STRING

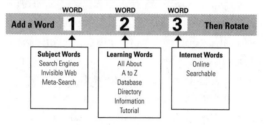

Select one word from each column and create a search string like this:

Search Engines Tutorial
Search Engines Directory
Invisible web tutorial
Invisible web online database

Then search on the words you selected. Study the results. Surf. Learn and enjoy what you find.

Then create another search string using different words and search again.

three

Magic Search Words

Most people don't know how to use a search engine. They typically use only one or two words. This yields very generalized, broad level information and often disappointing and frustrating results.

However, it doesn't have to be this way.

You get much, much better results if you use more words. In fact, if you use a carefully selected series or string of words, it can be magic.

Remember—MIMO = Magic In, Magic Out

The Search String Technique

Simple Searches

A simple search contains one or two words.

A "search string" is a series of words that you enter into a search engine. There is a first word, then a second word, then a third word, and so on.

<u>Word # 1 Word # 2 Word # 3 Word # 4 etc. . . .</u>

You can put in any series of words. You select the words to match the information you are looking for and want. Search strings contain the necessary words to find the Web site you need.

Remember, each time you add a word, the search engine looks through its database of indexed pages for Web sites that contain the words you have listed. The more words you list, the fewer Web pages will be found.

Whenever it finds a Web page with your query word on the page, it saves the URL or Web site address and brings it back to you with a list of pages where the word was found. The search engine actually brings back all the pages with your search word, sorted according to the Web site's criteria for *relevance.*

Each site's owner determines relevance by using factors such as word frequency, location of the search terms, relational clustering, link popularity, and good old pay-for-placement ranking. Generally, the more times the search word occurs, the higher on the list the Web page will be placed on the list. Voila!

A complex search, or a search string (which you will learn more about in a few pages), contains three, seven, perhaps as many as eleven carefully selected words.

Advanced Searches

Advanced searches use special terms (called Boolean terms or operators) to help you string together words to form a complex query and bring you back relevant results.

The most important advanced search terms are "AND", "OR", and "AND NOT".

It is important to read the instructions at any search engine you use. Each search engine operates according to its own set of rules. You must read the search engine instructions to understand what you will be getting when you do a search.

The default setting can be set to either AND or OR. If you search using two words with OR, the search engine brings back a lot more Web pages, that if you use the word AND.

This is because a search with two words and the default set to OR returns web pages containing either of your words. If the default setting is set to "AND", fewer pages will likely be found because both words will have to be present.

So if you want to get more sites on a topic, keep the search narrow, use the search term AND and don't use the search term OR.

At the time this book was written, the following default settings were in effect:

AND—Alta Vista, Excite, Fast, Google
OR—Hot Bot, Lycos, Northern Light

Many search engines allow you to substitute plus signs (+), spaces, and minus signs (-) for AND, OR, and AND NOT. Some, on the other hand, require you to use plus signs, spaces, and minus signs for AND, OR, and AND NOT.

Remember to read the instructions of the search engines you use.

There is a world of other advanced search options that various search engines use including things like:

Wild card truncations	Phrase searching
Automatic plurals	Stop words
Proximity searching	Field searching
Case sensitivity	

But for all but the most sophisticated and nerdy scientific users, you won't have to use these advanced search options.

And with the most popular search engines the technology is getting so good that you don't have to use the advanced search engine options unless you want to.

> You just enter your search words
> with a space between each word.

Explore the other search engine links and sites, so you can learn about search engines. Run the same search on other search engines.

In fact, at Google.com, you can do a search and then run the same key word searches on the other major search engines with just a click.

Concept and Phrase Searching

Here you simply turn a typical question or phrase into the actual words you use to search.

Phrase searching is very easy to use and can get you great results. Just take a simple question that you might say out loud to another person and turn it into a search string.

One powerful technique is to take a common phrase and add it to a *<Disease Word>* like the word "Diabetes" like this:

Coping with Diabetes

Run your search and evaluate your results.

Next, select a different phrase with your key search word, and search again, then evaluate results. You can continue until you achieve the information and understanding you are looking for on a specific subject.

Controlling Your Blood Sugar

You can continue till you achieve the information and understanding you are looking for on a certain subject.

The Minus Dot Com Trick

When you do a search and want to get past the hype associated with commercial Web sites, add the following words to your search string:

-.com.

Use this technique and watch the number of sites returned get reduced by almost half. This command will virtually eliminate the commercial sites and leave only the organizations (.org), education sites (.edu), and government sites (.gov) and military sites (.mil).

Let's show you how this is done.

Go to www.google.com and enter the word:

allergies

The response from the search engine reveals over 1,260,000 web sites. About half the links on the first page of search results are commercial companies that sell products. Some of these are great resources, but let's get rid of them anyway.

Now, let's do the minus dot com trick. Enter the words:

<u>allergies -.com</u>

The number of Web sites has dropped by two-thirds to just over 379,000 and the Web sites on the first page are from professional organizations and federal and state government agencies from the US and other English speaking countries. If you click on some of these links you will discover some of the best available information on the Internet on this subject very quickly.

So if you don't want to read through the commercial sites, use "The Minus Dot Com Technique".

<u><subject> –.com</u>

Similarly you can focus and zero in on certain types of sites by adding the search term ".org" or ".edu" or ".gov" or ".mil." like this.

<u>Word # 1 Word # 2 Word # 3 –.com .org</u>

There is one drawback from using the –.com technique. Many, many commercial sites are created and managed by experts, who give away an absolute ton of free, extremely high quality, high value educational information.

If you don't view commercial sites, you won't see these resources. But finding these requires you to use some more magic search words.

Magic Search "Learning Words"

There are a group of magic search words I call "Learning Words" which can be added to a subject search to help you zero in on some of these exquisite Web sites. You used one of them when you searched on the words "invisible Web tutorial".

The word *"tutorial"* is a magic search word. If you go to Merriam-Webster's Dictionary Online you will find it defined as:

> a paper, book, film, or computer program that provides practical information about a specific subject.

Pretty cool.

Free online tutorials produced by experts, as well as by universities, schools, government agencies are available on countless subjects of critical interest.

This one word can save you thousands and thousands of dollars in time, effort, and books.

Adding the word "tutorial" to a string of subject words can help locate expert information on nearly any topic quickly so you can learn what you need to know to take your next steps.

Try the following searches:

<u>alternative medicine tutorial</u>
<u>human body tutorial</u>
<u>choosing a doctor tutorial</u>
<u>choosing health insurance tutorial</u>
<u>senior long term care facility tutorial</u>

There are several other critical magic "Learning Words" you can use to find more critical information.

A to Z	Guide
All About	Index
Ask a Doctor	Introduction
Ask an Expert	Library
Ask the Professional	List
Database	Manual
Dictionaries	Patient information
Directory	

One major sub-category of *<Learning Words>* is "free" stuff.

The word "free" is, by itself, a powerful magic word. Use it as soon as you encounter information requiring payment. Add it to your search strings frequently.

You find the free stuff by searching on the following words:

Advice	Do's and don'ts
Book	E-mail consultations
Booklet	Forum
Bulletin board	Guide

Help

Help centers

Manual

Online manual

Quiz

Self help

Strategies

Tactics

Test

Tips

Tutorial

Magic Search "Internet Words"

You will open up additional doors to more valuable Web sites if you also use these words with another category of magic search words called "Internet Words".

These are the words that have developed since the Internet was created and became a uniquely commercialized advertising and marketing telecommunications medium.

The key magical "Internet Words" to use in search strings include:

Bank

Central

Clearinghouse

Gateway

Interactive

Jumpstation

Learning center

Link

Market

Multimedia

Network

Online

Resource center

Searchable

Specialized

Supersite

Virtual

These words are often used in the name of a Web site or in the first paragraph describing the Web site. So when you search with these words, they easily bring back these Web sites.

Now combine these two techniques and see what sort of magic occurs.

Try some of the following searches:

medical health online database

medical information directories

patient information searchable directories

medical health resource center

You can narrow these searches by adding a special subject or topic like this:

<u>*<disease word>* searchable online database</u>
<u>*<medical issue>* online database</u>

Example:

<u>Staph infection searchable online database</u>

You will learn more about how to select additional search terms to zero in on medical topics and issues that are in your particular areas of interest in the next section.

Special Tactics for Creating Search Strings

Creating Search Strings

We've discussed both search engines and the types of searches. At this point, your goal is to find Web sites that contain the certain types of information that will satisfy your wants and desires. Now, what is left to discuss is the "how"—how do you find these Web sites?

You create a search word string (or a search string for short). You slowly and carefully string together a series of words.

Search strings contain the necessary magic search words to find the Web sites you need, and you create these search word strings systematically, one word at a time.

1. ADD A WORD

Remember, a search string is a series of magic search words that you enter into a search engine. There is a first word, then a second word, then a third word, and so on.

<u>Word # 1 Word # 2 Word # 3 Word # 4</u>

And so on.

You can put in any series of words. Your choice of words is based entirely on what you are looking to find.

But what words do you pick?

You pick the magic search words that will open up the best sources of information on the Internet.

This book is all about finding medical health information, so let's start right at the beginning and learn how to do that.

Go to www.google.com and enter the words

<u>medical health information</u>
<u>women's health information</u>
<u>men's health information</u>
<u>diseases symptoms treatments a to z</u>
<u>Types of disease list</u>

You can get a lot of basic information about general health topics by doing these and other simple *<phrase word>* searches.

You will find specialized Web sites created by commercial entities as well as professional organizations, government agencies, media and experts from all over the world. But you can do better than this.

2. SEARCH STRING WORD GROUPS

You start searching by selecting words that describe what you want to find. Selecting the best magic search words and getting the best results often means experimenting with different but related words. These words form the *search string word group*.

A *search string word group* contains the key word as well as **synonyms** that mean the same thing, or other related words that are similar in meaning and can be just as useful to you.

What this means is that a word or its synonyms or other similar related words are all useful magic search words that can be used to find high-value Web sites.

How do you find synonyms? You search of course. Search on the words:

<u>synonyms</u>

Or on the related words

<u>online thesaurus</u>

You will find numerous free online sources that can be used to identify synonyms and related magic search words. You can always apply some plain old thinking and common sense. Related words will come to you quite readily whenever you ponder a challenge and need to come up with a word to embark on a search.

There are several other key search string word groups that are especially useful for finding health information. These are:

<Disease Words>	<Family Words>
<Anatomy Words>	<Internet Words>
<Body Part Words>	<Learning Words>
<Medical Action Words>	<Industry Words>
<Medical Specialty Words>	<Association Words>
<Medical Issue Words>	<Location Words>
<Symptom Words>	<Source Words>
<Age Words>	<Media Words>
<Gender Words>	<Time Words>
<Country or Culture Words>	

There are many more search string word groups you will think up as you identify and pursue your particular and unique needs. We'll talk about these in more detail later.

When you create a search string use the "add a word" technique. Select one magic search word from one key search string word group and then add another magic search word from another word group and so on and so on. Think of this as a Chinese menu, where you just take one item from column A, then one item from column B, and so on.

You vary your word selection to meet your needs. You add words in sequence, with a specific purpose, one word at a time so that your search results bring you back results—Web pages that contain the words you seek.

Then, you evaluate the results of your search.

Obviously, this will take time. But, it will be worth your time and effort if you go through this process.

Start at the beginning with your most general search and conduct one search after the other, reading and evaluating the results along the way, as you work though a short list of the search words.

Here is an example:

Goal: Identifying a free online expert to answer questions about allergy treatments for children.

Follow along and pay careful attention as we build this search string together. Open your browser and go to your favorite search engine. Either enter what is presented below, or enter your own personal interests and information. The underlined words are the words you add at each step.

1. First you enter the magic search words that contain a *<Disease Word>.*

Allergies

2. Then you add a *<Medical Action Word>.*

Allergies **treatment**

3. Add two *<Internet Words>.*

Allergies treatment **free online**

4. Add some *<Learning Words>.*

Allergies treatment free online **ask an expert**

5. Add an *<Age Word>.*

Allergies treatment free online ask an expert **kids**

As you construct the search string, take a look at the list of Web sites your search brings, step by step.

Click on a couple of the sites and see what kinds of information they contain, but don't spend too much time on each sequential step. Go back to the search form page and continue to add words. Work your way through to the end and create the eight-word search string.

This table illustrates how each magic search word is associated with a search string word group.

Search word	Word Group	Example
Word 1	Disease Word	Allergies
Word 2	Medical Action Word	Treatment
Word 3	Internet Words	Free Online
Word 4	Learning Words	Ask an Expert
Word 5	Age Word	Kids

Wow. You nailed it. You found what you were looking for. Web sites with free expert questions and answers covering allergy treatments for children. Pretty amazing.

For those of you reading along, assume that you have executed the search, evaluated your results by clicking on some of the more promising sites.

Now, we're going to introduce a new technique that will open up a whole new world of possibilities with just one click.

3. SEARCH WORD ROTATION

Let's say you searched on the words:

<u>High blood pressure symptoms</u>

High blood pressure is your *<Disease Word>*.

You want to find out more information about high blood pressure only this time you want to learn about "causes". The word "causes" is a *<Medical Action Word>*, that is, it describes the type of special information, help or assistance, or guidance you are looking for. Notice it is an important, operative, action-laden word.

What you do is simply substitute one magic search word in the search string to focus your search on those other types of *<Medical Action Words>*.

<u>High blood pressure **causes**</u>

Now ask yourself, "What other types of special information about this disease am I interested in?"

Here is a list of other important *<Medical Action Words>*:

Alternatives	Rehabilitation
Cause	Symptoms
Diagnosis	Treatment
Medication	Therapy
Prevention	

Now use the "search word rotation" technique. What you do is rotate or substitute just one word, in this case, the key *<Medical Action Word>* with another of the *<Medical Action Words>* on your list. The search again to find Web sites that contain these words and represent new sources of crucial information.

You rotate the search words like this:

Search 1 = High blood pressure *control*

Search 2 = High blood pressure *prevention*

Search 3 = High blood pressure *treatment alternatives*

Search 4 = High blood pressure *medications*

Search 5 = High blood pressure *medication side effects*

This is very powerful. So take your time.

You can rotate the magic search words in your search string with synonyms or similar words for any word you select and continue to find more new and different Web sites.

You can rotate using the **synonyms** for the *<Disease Word>* or on any of the *<Medical Action Words>* or on any other word in your search string. You use the synonyms and related words in the appropriate word group.

Remember each time you do this, rotate just one word and retain the remainder of the original string of magic search words, keeping all the other words in the search string the same. Make only one change at a time. Be slow and systematic and you will gain tremendous comprehensive knowledge and understanding of the disease or issue you are interested in.

This is actually a really great exercise for you to do on your computer, so you can see just how powerful a tool you now have at your fingertips.

You can use this technique to find scholarships, jobs, health information, legal advice, or just about anything.

The selective addition and rotation of words allows you to take advantage of the incredible power of search engine technology.

Each additional word opens up an entirely new, but equally detailed, set of search results. And all you did was add one word to your search.

Think of the possibilities! You can use magic search words, create all sorts of search strings, and rotate through a whole new universe of different areas of knowledge, opportunity, and interest.

Congratulations. If you use these techniques, you can now explore the realm of possibility like never before.

4. SEARCH BY AGE, EDUCATION OR GENDER

You can select and rotate magic search words to focus your search for specific health information that pertains to people of a certain age or gender.

<Age Words>

Babies
Infants
Toddlers
Teens
Parents
Young adults
Adults
Single
Married
Divorced
Mature adults
Middle age
Retired
Seniors
Mature
Elderly

K–12
Middle school
Private school
Vocational
Technical
Associate
Two Year
Four year
Community College
College
University
Bachelors
Masters
Graduate
Post graduate
Doctoral
Postdoctoral

<Education Words>

Students
Elementary school
High school
Teachers
Parents
K–6

<Gender Words>

Girls
Boys
Male
Female
Man
Woman

5. SEARCH BY LOCATION

You can add a city, county, state, region or country to your search string and then systematically search city by city through places you are interested in like this:

nursing homes **Los Angeles California**

Then you can rotate through other locations quickly like this:

<u>nursing homes</u> **San Diego California**
<u>nursing homes</u> **Los Angeles California**
<u>nursing homes</u> **Miami Florida**
<u>nursing homes</u> **Tampa Florida**

Geography and location can be used to effectively to pinpoint facilities, services, physicians or other support service providers or opportunities with many of the search string word groups. Use your hometown as a *<Location Word>* in your search strings to get detailed information about information and service providers in your local area.

6. SEARCH BY DATE

You can eliminate Web sites that are outdated by adding the current or upcoming year to your search string like this:

<u>rehabilitation counseling patient information</u> **2002**

However, don't be too hasty in doing this. Many Web sites don't change information every year, and the inclusion of the year or date will eliminate many sites that may interest you.

7. SEARCHING FOR SPECIFIC SOURCES OF INFORMATION

You can focus your search *<Information Source Words>* to specifically focus on the information provided by different types of institutions, government agencies, companies, professional health or medical associations or organizations.

Government

City, county, state, regional, and federal government agencies

Companies & Corporations

Companies by name
Companies by industry

Associations

Professional and trade associations

Professional and trade organizations
Nonprofit organizations
Philanthropic foundations, Institutions
Trade groups
Fraternal organizations
Community organizations

Educational Institutions

Schools, Colleges, Universities

Each of these is a key search word group that has specific terminology that is best used when searching the Internet. You simply add a source word to your search string like this:

<u>medication heart problems</u> **drug companies**
<u>selecting medical doctors guidance</u> **associations**
<u>medical devices</u> **government**

The later chapters of this book provide special techniques and the magic search words and terminology to use in searching the sources of medical and health information.

8. SEARCH THE MEDIA (PRINT AND ELECTRONIC)

Most media have Web sites on the Internet. You start by finding media on the Internet by creating a search string using the magic words Media *<Learning Words> <Internet Words>* like this:

<u>media online directory</u>
<u>media online database</u>

Next, use the add a word technique to isolate the type of media you are interested in:

Daily newspapers	Magazines
Weekly newspapers	Trade publications
News services	Radio
News syndicates	Television

Search for specific media by location either by state or city and state. Finally, once you are on a Web site for a specific media publication, search that site for the information you seek.

Media tend to have what we described earlier as "invisible Web" resources. To gain access to those resources you must first go to the Web site, then locate the entrance to search tools. After locating the directories, searchable databases and libraries, you can follow the instructions and use the resources.

For example search on the following words:

<u>daily newspapers New York</u>

Then search for one of the newspapers you find. It could be The New York Times, The Wall Street Journal, or Newsday.

Once you get to the media's Web site, then search on the words "health" and your *<Disease Words>* or other topics of interest.

At newspapers and magazines you will find articles about the subjects you are interested in. At professional journals you will find peer reviewed technical articles.

Try the following searches:

<u>Magazines medical health A to Z</u>
<u>Magazines parenting online</u>
<u>Trade journals environmental medicine</u>
<u>TV shows health medical</u>
<u>Radio shows women's health</u>

More and more media organizations are going online and they will give you searchable database or directory access to their archives. Some are for free while others are accessible for a fee.

9. USE CONCEPT OR PHRASE SEARCHING

Simple Phrase Searching

Here, you turn a typical question or phrase into the actual words you use to search.

Phrase searching is easy to use and can get you great results. Just take a simple question that you might say out loud to another person and turn it into a search string.

One powerful technique is to take a common phrase and add it to a *<Disease Word>*. Run your search and evaluate your results.

Select a different phrase with your *<Disease Word>*, and search again, then evaluate results. You can continue till you achieve the information and understanding you are looking for on a certain subject.

The search string construction looks like this:

<u><phrase> <Disease Word></u>
<u><phrase> <Disease word> <Medical Action Word></u>

There are lots of phrases that you can use:

An introduction to

Avoiding the problem of

Coping with

Dealing With

Healthy Living

How to

Keeping healthy

Keeping strong

Keeping well

Living with

Managing for

Planning for

Protecting against

Risks to human health from

Surviving with

The best techniques for

The biggest mistakes

The role of

Tips on preventing

Treating the

Understanding how to

Want to know more? *<Disease Word>*

Want to know more? *<Medical Issue Word>*

What to do if

What to do when

When you have

When you have to

Here are some examples:

<u>What to do when your wife is having a baby</u>
<u>Managing your medication</u>
<u>Managing your cholesterol</u>
<u>Surviving you heart attack</u>
<u>The biggest nutrition mistakes athletes make</u>
<u>How to treat your gum disease</u>
<u>Avoiding the problem of diabetic foot disease</u>
<u>Risks to human health from work</u>
<u>Healthy Living Thyroid</u>

More Detailed Phrase Searching

You can use more detailed phrase searching by adding more search string word groups to your phrase. For example, to find information to help family members, the search string construction is this:

<phrase> <Disease Word> <Personal Relation> <Action Word>

You enter the phrase with the words from any other search string word groups you wish to research.

Mothers of *<Disease Word>*
Fathers of *<Disease Word>*
When your *<Personal Relation>* has *<Disease Word>*
How to protect your *<Family Member>* from *<Disease Word>*
How to help your *<Family Member>* overcome *<Health Problem>*
Here are some examples:

mothers of asthmatics
when your mother has alzheimer's disease
when your husband has porn addition
when your father is dying of cancer
what should i do about <health problem>?
what should you do if you have <health problem>?
how to protect your children from drugs
how to help your teenager deal with peer pressure drinking
dealing with stigma from mentally ill relative
specific resume problems
overcoming career problems
finding a better job
job and career fair resources

10. EXACT QUOTE SEARCHING

This technique is useful when you are looking for an exact book title or an article about something specific.

With some search engines you enter the exact sequence of words you want to use with quotation marks around them.

Other search engines have you enter the words in a special text box.

In any case, you should refer to and use the advanced search engine instructions that you find on the particular search engine you are using.

Here are some examples:

"dealing with heart disease"
"living with aids"
"dealing with dying"
"coping with irritable bowel syndrome"
"when your child has asthma"
"planning for your pregnancy"

You can also use exact quote searching to find specific medical facilities, schools, or universities, or government agencies or professional organizations.

Examples:

"Kennewick General Hospital"
"Lourdes Health Network"
"Kadlec Medical Center"
"American Medical Association"
"Centers for Disease Control"

Some search engines consider some words to be so common that they are ignored. These are typically called "stop words." If you read the advanced search engine instructions, you can find a way around this. Google, for example, will let you include a "stop word" if you place a "plus sign" in front of the stop word, like this:

Plastic surgeons preferred providers +with offices in Seattle

You may get very few results by using exact quote searching, but you will likely get exactly what you asked for.

11. SEARCH FOR INFORMATION IN DIFFERENT LANGUAGES

Information is available on the Internet from a wide variety of countries all over the world, in numerous languages.

You can enter your search in the language you are seeking to find the information.

You can also enter your search in English and add the specific language you are seeking.

Example:

<u>AIDS/HIV Information bilingual</u>
<u>AIDS/HIV Resource Centers Spanish</u>

You can also search for the country you are looking for.
Example:

<u>Diabetes Patient Information England</u>
<u>Migraine Treatment Australia</u>

You can also search for Web sites that are located in a certain country by entering the URL country code:

<u>migraine information France French .fr</u>
<u>medical information Russia .ru</u>

Find Internet country codes by conducting a search using the magic words:

Internet country codes

Some search engines allow you to select Web sites that contain the selected language you want. For example, go to www.Google.com, and select your desired language in the preferences setting.

Magic Search Words Roadmap

The following chart illustrates how to select magic search words to create search strings using the word groups discussed in the chapter.

Practice the basic search skills

First open up your favorite search engine. My favorite is www.Google.com, but you may like another. It doesn't matter which one you like the best.

Magic Search Words
HEALTH
CREATE A SEARCH STRING

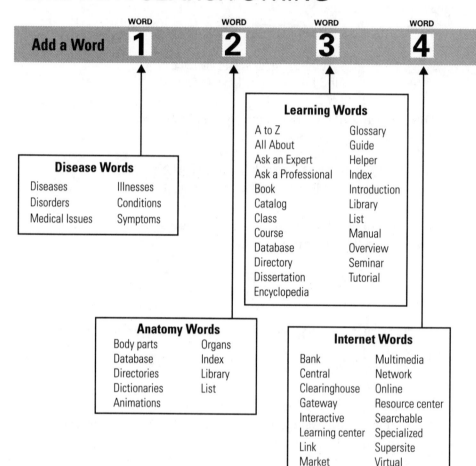

Add a Word

| WORD 1 | WORD 2 | WORD 3 | WORD 4 |

Learning Words

A to Z	Glossary
All About	Guide
Ask an Expert	Helper
Ask a Professional	Index
Book	Introduction
Catalog	Library
Class	List
Course	Manual
Database	Overview
Directory	Seminar
Dissertation	Tutorial
Encyclopedia	

Disease Words

Diseases	Illnesses
Disorders	Conditions
Medical Issues	Symptoms

Anatomy Words

Body parts	Organs
Database	Index
Directories	Library
Dictionaries	List
Animations	

Internet Words

Bank	Multimedia
Central	Network
Clearinghouse	Online
Gateway	Resource center
Interactive	Searchable
Learning center	Specialized
Link	Supersite
Market	Virtual

Search Engines

True Search Engines   Invisible Web

Virtual Libraries   Directories   Metasearch

Concept &
Phrase Searches

The Minus .com Trick
-.com

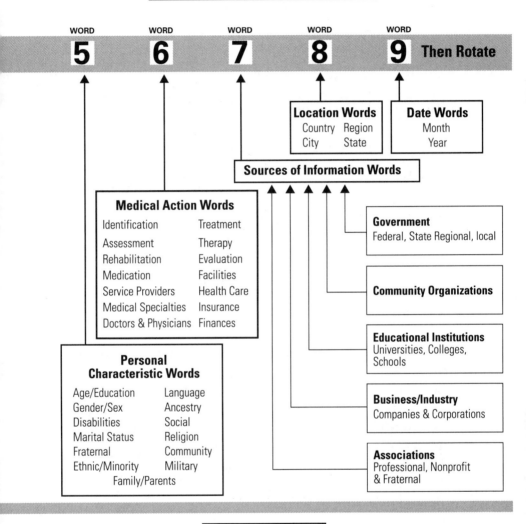

Action Plan

Look for Critical Business Information (CBI)
Then search, find, match and apply!

WORD **5** WORD **6** WORD **7** WORD **8** WORD **9** **Then Rotate**

Location Words
Country Region
City State

Date Words
Month
Year

Sources of Information Words

Government
Federal, State Regional, local

Medical Action Words

Identification	Treatment
Assessment	Therapy
Rehabilitation	Evaluation
Medication	Facilities
Service Providers	Health Care
Medical Specialties	Insurance
Doctors & Physicians	Finances

Community Organizations

Educational Institutions
Universities, Colleges,
Schools

Personal Characteristic Words

Age/Education	Language
Gender/Sex	Ancestry
Disabilities	Social
Marital Status	Religion
Fraternal	Community
Ethnic/Minority	Military
Family/Parents	

Business/Industry
Companies & Corporations

Associations
Professional, Nonprofit
& Fraternal

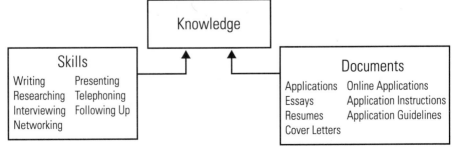

Knowledge

Skills

Writing	Presenting
Researching	Telephoning
Interviewing	Following Up
Networking	

Documents

Applications	Online Applications
Essays	Application Instructions
Resumes	Application Guidelines
Cover Letters	

Then, read the next section looking for something that interests you.

Once you find what you are interested in, create a search string using the search words that you want to use. Keep your search strings simple and focus on one area of interest at a time to start:

<u>teenagers depression</u>

Then make them more targeted

<u>teenagers depression **support centers New York**</u>

Then use the search word rotation technique with synonyms and related words.

Or if you want to find a psychological counselor nearby where you live and you are in Spokane, Washington enter the words:

<u>Psychological counselors Spokane Washington</u>

Then use the search word rotation technique with synonyms and related words.

Make sure you search with various *<Internet Words>* and *<Learning Words>*.

Search using various *<Information Source Words>*.

Finally, switch to a new subject and start over again.

We'll teach you to get more systematic and comprehensive about searching for medical health information in the next section.

For now, just play with what you've learned so far.

Got it? Now turn on your computer.

Ready? Get set.

Go!

four

The Magic Search Words Kingdom

It is crucial to see the big picture and understand that what you are doing when you search for medical health information on the Internet. You are using magic search words to search out power in the universe. Words have magic. They lead you to information. Information gives you power. Power enables you to take action. Action allows you to realize benefits.

The better the magic search words, the better the information you find, the more powerful you will become.

Overview of the Kingdom

Work through this next section slowly and carefully to clearly understand and master how to use these procedures. You are going to learn how to select magic search words from six major realms of technology and knowledge.

Each realm contains several key search string word groups. Pay attention to how these are organized because they form a framework for searching that will become a powerful tool for you to use.

The six realms are:

1. **The Internet itself:** You take advantage of the terminology and technology the Internet offers. We introduced this when we showed you all about search engines and how they work. You already know how to use the Magic Search Words for uncovering high quality educational information. These are:
   - Learning Words
   - Internet Words

2. **The science of health and medicines**: You search for specific disease information and medical help and guidance and other forms of expert using the language and terminology of the science:
   - Human Anatomy Words
     a. Body Part Words
     b. Organ Systems
     c. Cellular biology
   - Disease Words
   - Symptom Words
   - Medical Action Words
   - Medical Specialty Words
   - Medical Issue Words

3. **Your personal characteristics and wants**: You identify and recognize who you are and what you want, e.g., your qualifications, characteristics and interests:
   - Personal and Social Characteristic Words
   - Age Words
   - Gender Words
   - Family Words
   - Culture Words

4. **The Key Sources of Information**: You search for the specific sources of medical information:
   - Government
   - Medical facilities

- Universities, colleges, and schools
- Professional Medical Organizations
- Professional and nonprofit associations
- Companies and corporations
- Community organizations

5. **Other Personal Needs or Desires**: You adjust your search to meet other personal needs or desires:
   - Location
   - Time

6. **The Media**: You also search for information that will provide you with additional information and possible sources of knowledge and contacts.
   - Newspapers and Magazines
   - Radio
   - TV

When you create search strings, the Magic Search Words you will use come from the Key Search String Word Groups contained in each of the six realms.

Magic Potions: The Key Search Word String Word Groups

This section contains a mid-level look at the types of magic search words that you can use in the actual search strings you create. The next section drops down to one more level of detail to give you even more specific search string recipes.

Three Specific Goals for Searching

You select search words to achieve three specific all-important objectives:

1. Increase your knowledge of a specific health or medical topic.
2. Identify specific alternative treatments or remedies or other actions that you can choose to utilize or make a decision about.
3. Improve your skills, abilities and success in selecting, dealing with and effectively managing the medical professionals or facilities you interact with, and getting better care or treatment.

When you create search strings you aim at satisfying your information needs in one of these areas.

You use the search string word groups to guide your selection of the right magic search words each time you do a search to achieve your objectives.

Inside the Key Medical Search String Word Groups

Below each word group listed here you will find important magic search words you can use to create search strings.

\<Learning Words\>

A to Z	Latest News
Chronic	Layperson
Database	Library
Definition of Terms	Manual
Dictionary	Online
Directory	Outbreaks
Encyclopedia	PDQ (Physicians Data Query)
Glossary	Searchable Databases
Introduction	Terminology
Issues	Terms
Index	Topics

The starting search string construction looks like this:

<u>\<Disease Words\> \<Learning Word\></u>

or

<u>\<Medical Issue Word\> \<Learning Word\></u>

Each of these will lead you to Web sites that can offer up a wide spectrum of information on diseases from the lay person to the most technical.

Remember this is powerful magic you are using. Use it wisely.

Here are some examples:

Alphabetical index diseases illnesses conditions directory alphabetical index human health

centers for disease control and prevention

CDC disease directory

CDC disease database

diseases a to z

diseases conditions index list

diseases glossary

directory of diseases

databases of diseases

genetic disorders index

illnesses glossary

infectious diseases a to z

infectious diseases directory

CDC disease outbreaks latest news

medical health conditions a to z

medical health databases

medical encyclopedia

medical health disorders dictionary

medical disorders a to z

medical health library

medical health manual

medical health searchable
  databases

medical health dictionary

medicine health online dictionary

medical procedures index

medical health tests index

medical equipment index

medical terminology dictionary

medical terms index

patient education center <disease>

patient FAQ's (frequently asked
  questions)

patient information <Disease Word>

patient resources <Disease Word>

patient treatment documents
  <Disease Word>

This simple and powerful search string that can be improved by adding an *<Internet Word>*

<Medical Issue Word> <Learning Word> <Internet Word>

Here are some examples:

medical disorders a to z online directory
medical health virtual library
medical health online manual
medical health searchable online databases
medical health online dictionary
medicine health online dictionary

<Human Anatomy Words>

There is a mind-boggling amount of free information on the Internet concerning human anatomy and the parts of your body. The magic search words in his particular area of science allow you to receive a state of the art education like nothing you have ever seen or imagined.

To get a general education and find highly colorful instructive, interactive and multi-media Web sites create search strings using some of the following:

<Anatomy Words>

Animations inner body
Body atlas online
Cross sections
Databases
Free illustrated guides
Free online guides
Graphics anatomy
Gray's Anatomy online
Images

Interactive Human Body Online
Multi-media
Online Exploration
Pictures
Science guides
Three dimensional imagery
Tutorial
Virtual Human Body
Whole body viewers

Here are some examples:

human body animations
human anatomy interactive online
body maps multimedia
visible human project
human body diagrams images
microscopic images interactive
anatomy databases
virtual human body
human biology tutorial

<Body Part Words>

You can zero in and learn about specific parts of your body by identifying the specific body part using the following search words. Do some phrase searches:

Learn your body parts
Human anatomy list
Human *<body part word>* information
Human *<body part word>* *<Learning Word>*
Human *<body part word>* dissections index

Here is a list of specific *<body part words>*:

skeleton	muscles
bones	circulatory system
nervous system	genetics
organs	

You can just as easily switch your area of interest from human beings of any age or gender to pets or animals. Just use the magic search words that focus your search on your favorite furry friend:

pets	animal care
animals	veterinary care
pet care	<specific animal>

<Cellular Biology>

Cellular biology is an important aspect of medicine and health. If you have a disease and need to interact with your physician the more you know about cellular biology the greater your understanding will be.

You can learn a lot very quickly by searching on the words *<Cellular Biology>* with the following magic search words:

Basic tutorial	Online
Introduction	Virtual library
Dictionary	Interactive
Information resource	

You can also conduct some *<Phrase Word>* Searches:

Inside a Cell

Tissues and Organs

Parts of a Cell

How Cells Reproduce

<Organ System Words>

Organ systems are another important aspect of medicine and health. You can learn a lot by searching on the specific *<Organ System Word>* you are interested in:

Cardiovascular	Nervous
Respiratory	Skin

Musculoskeletal
Blood
Digestive
Endocrine

Urinary
Male reproductive
Female reproductive

<Phrase and concept searches>

You can also conduct some *<phrase and concept searches>*:

all about your digestive system
learn about your cardiovascular system
understand your reproductive system

<Disease Words>

The key synonyms in this all important search string word group are:

Diseases
Illnesses
Disorders
Conditions

You can use these interchangeably or appropriately as you find it used in the field, based on your particular need or circumstance.

To find the name of a specific disease, search on the words:

Diseases <Learning Words>
Diseases <Learning Words> <Internet Words>

Like this:

diseases a to z
diseases directory
diseases database
diseases online searchable database

Once you locate a specialized directory or database, look up your specific disease or disorder of concern.

Here are other searches that are useful in getting to specific disease information:

<u><disease> quick reference</u>
<u><medical specialty> quick reference</u>
<u><disease> online medical dictionaries layperson</u>
<u><disease> online medical information simplified</u>
<u><disease> online medical reference guide simplified</u>
<u><disease> online consultation</u>

<Symptom Words>

To find the name for what ails you or to identify the specific medical or health issue you are interested in, you may have to first identify the symptoms.

Use *<Symptom Words>* to help identify specific diseases, or identify appropriate treatments. The search word construction would be:

<u><body part><symptom words> <diagnosis></u>
<u><disease><symptom><diagnosis></u>

Here is a very special magic search word string will get you to some of the most incredible specialized searchable databases ever created, all available online for free. These databases can help you self-diagnose your disease. Search on the words

<u>Diseases symptoms diagnosis online</u>

In many cases you will prefer to zero in on the actual symptom that plagues you and use this specific symptom word with a *<medical action word>* like this:

<u><Symptom Word> <Medical Action Word></u>

Example:

<u>stomach pain diagnosis</u>
<u>stomach pain treatment</u>

Here is a detailed list of *<Symptom Words>*:

Aches and pains	Back Pain
Aching	Bleeding

Bloating

Bone pain

Broken

Cold

Constipation

Coughing

Diarrhea

Discoloration

Dryness

Farting

Fever

Fractures

Heavy mucus production

Hot

Inflammation

Injured

Intestinal gas

Irritation pain

Itchy eyes

Lumps

Nasal congestion

Odor

Pain

Pain

Raspy throat

Red

Red eyes

Respiratory failure

Serious injury

Shivering

Skin rashes

Smell

Sneezes

Sniffles

Sore

Splotchy

Sprains

Strains

Stuffed Nose

Swelling

Swollen

Tenderness

Torn

Ulcers

Vomiting

Wheezing

<Medical Action Words>

You have a disease, an illness, a disorder, or a condition and need to know how to deal with it. The *<Medical Action Word>* describes the type of help or assistance or information you are looking for:

The most common *<Medical Action Words>* are:

Symptoms

Diagnosis

Cause

Prevention

Treatment

Medication

Therapy

Rehabilitation

Here is a more thorough list of medical action words to use with disease or illness searches

Alternatives

Assessment

Causes

Control

Diagnosis

Education

Effects

Emergencies

Help

Hospital Care

Identification

Immunizations

Impacts

Implants

Incidence

Medications

Prevention

Prognosis

Rehabilitation

Replants

Risk Factors

Screening

Self Help

Side Effects

Support

Surgery

Symptoms

Therapy

Transplants

Treatment

X-rays

You conduct searches by using the following search string:

<Disease Word> and a <Medical Action Word>

Examples:

food allergies diagnosis
back pain prevention
chronic disease treatment
sore throat medications
acne prevention treatment

These search strings will quickly bring you to helpful information that you can use to increase your understanding and evaluate further options.

Remember to use the Minus Dot Com Trick to reduce the risks of incorrect or less than complete and accurate information from commercial or alternative web sites by focusing on governmental, professional, or bona fide medical university sources of information.

<Doctor & Medical Specialty Words>

Often you will want to search for information about the particular branch of medicine or identify the specific type of doctors that specialize in a certain area of medicine. The following search words are useful:

ask about <disease>

medical specialties index
medical specialties a to z
medical specialties layperson explanation
virtual medical library medical specialties

You can do some phrases searches:

ask about <disease>
ask an expert <disease>
ask the experts <disease>
ask a professional <disorder>
ask the professionals <disorder>
ask the doctor <sex>
call a <doctor specialty>

Examples:

ask a doctor woman
diabetes disorder online consultation
ask an expert male menopause
hypertension reference guide simplified
ask about cancer

Locating a Doctor:

You can locate or identify doctors by searching using the following search words:

find a doctor <illness>
find a dentist <location>
find a surgeon <specialty>
online <medical specialty> consultation
physician locator <specialty>
physician locator <disease>

You can target your search for specific medical specialists geographically by adding in a *<Location Word>*.

Example:

physical therapist Aspen Colorado

<Medical Specialty or Discipline Words>

You can search for and learn about specific medical specialties by name:

Allergists & Immunologists
Anesthesiologists
Cardiologists Colon & Rectal
   Surgeons
Dermatologists
Emergency Medicine Specialists
Endocrinologists
Family Practitioners (FPs)
Gastroenterologists
General Practitioners (GPs)
Geriatric Specialists
Hematologists
Infectious Disease Specialists
Internists (IMs)
Nephrologists
Neurological Surgeons
Neurologists
Nuclear Medicine Specialists
Obstetricians & Gynecologists

Oncologists
Ophthalmologists
Orthopedic Surgeons
Otalaryngologists
Pathologists
Pediatricians
Physical Medicine and
   Rehabilitation Specialists
Plastic Surgeons
Preventive Medicine Specialists
Psychiatrists
Pulmonologists
Radiologists
Rheumatologists
Sports Medicine Specialists
Surgeons (General)
Thoracic Surgeons
Urologists
Vascular Surgeons

<Age, Gender, Family & Culture Words>

You narrow and better define the type of medical or health information you find by using *<Age, Gender, Family & Culture Words>* in your search strings.

The search string construction looks like this:

<age><Disease><action desired>
<gender><Disorder><action desired>
<family relation><condition><medical action word>
<ethnicity><Disease><medical action word>
<age> <Body Part><Disease><medical action word>

Here are specific *<Age, Gender, Family & Culture Words>*:

<Age Words>

Newborns
Infants

Children   Seniors

Teens   Matures

Students   Elderly

Adults

Examples:

<u>newborn hearing problems detection</u>

<u>infants sudden death prevention</u>

<u>children mouth injuries protection</u>

<u>students drug testing legal rights</u>

<u>elderly physical abuse identification</u>

\<Gender Words\>

Male   Women

Female   Girls

Men   Boys

Examples:

<u>male menopause symptoms diagnosis</u>

<u>female depression prevention management</u>

<u>girls sexual abuse education</u>

<u>teenagers preventing sports injuries</u>

\<Family Relation Words\>

Parents   Aunt

Father   Uncle

Mother   Cousin

Brother   Grandmother

Sister   Grandfather

Examples:

<u>my father is an alcoholic</u>

<u>mother has breast cancer</u>

<u>brother is drug addict</u>

<u>grandfather has diabetes</u>

<u>my teenager is pregnant</u>

\<Culture Words\>

You can find information that is specific to a given social group, ethnic group or country by searching on those terms. The magic search words to use include:

Country of origin   Ethnic culture
Country of interest   Minority group
Cultural group of origin

Examples:

<u>Jewish genetic disorders</u>
<u>African AIDS prevention</u>
<u>Chinese acupuncture treatment</u>
<u>Native American Indian disease incidence</u>
<u>Japan recipes nutritional content</u>

Magic Spells: Selecting the Magic Search Words

This section summarizes the key search tactics. Remember you are selecting individual magic search words from each word group like a Chinese menu. Start simple. First create simple search strings and evaluate your results. Then make more complex search strings by adding words from other search string word groups.

Key Search Strings

There are several search strings that you will use again and again because they provide excellent information quickly in any area of health or medicine that you may be interested in. The best search strings are summarized below, along with a mini-road map illustrating the magic search word sequence you can use.

<Disease Word> <Learning Word> <Internet Word>

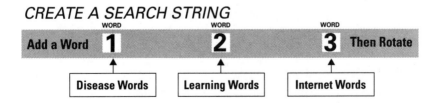

Decide What You Want

The first step in creating your search string is to identify exactly what you are looking for. Be as narrow and specific as you can possibly be. The first word of your search string should always be a *<Disease Words>* or a *<Medical Issue Word>* or a *<Medical Specialty Word>* or a subject that you are interested in.

Add any and all the other words you select from specific search word groups to these *<subject words>* like this:

<u><Disease Words> plus the rest of your search string</u>

To be successful in your search you must have some ideas as to what you want, what will satisfy you, and what information sources you will trust.

Focus on what you can read easily and understand readily. Your searching should be enjoyable. The information you find should be something that you will be happy with. Look for what interests you.

Be specific and careful about what you seek.

Remember to try to qualify the quality of the information by noting the source of the information. Is it an alternative health source? Is it a government agency? Is it a medical university? How trustworthy is the information? Try to find out.

You can get exactly what you ask for if you try. You can find exactly what you want.

Building the Best Health Search Strings

While there are lots of possible combinations, the best search strings use Magic Search Words from just a few of the important search string word groups. They include the following:

<Disease Words> <Learning Word> <Internet Word>
<Medical Issue Word> <Learning Word> <Internet Word>
<Disease Word> <Medical Action Word> <Symptom Word>
<Medical Issue Word> <Medical Action Word> <Symptom Word>

<Disease Words> <Anatomy Word> <Learning Word> <Internet Word>
<Disease Word> <Anatomy Word> <Medical Action Word> <Symptom Word>

Using these three to four word group search stings is a very powerful search technique. The use of these search strings makes researching specific medical and health topics very simple.

Simple Medical Health Search Strings

Search by entering a *<Disease Word>* and a *<Medical Action Word>*
  Example:

breast cancer diagnosis

headache treatment

broken bone therapy

heart healthy eating

post operation rehabilitation

CREATE A SEARCH STRING

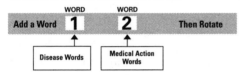

Complex Medical Health Search Strings

Get a little more specific by creating search strings by adding words from two or more search string word groups:

  Create search strings by selecting words from each relevant search string words group. Try to use one word from two, then three, then four then five groups and so on.

<Learning Words>   <Symptom Word>

<Internet Words>   <Medical Specialty Word>

<Anatomy Words>   <Medical Action Word>

<Body Part Words>   <Age, Sex, Family & Culture Word>

<Disease Word>

The search string construction is like this:

<Body part> <Disease> <Medical action word>
<Disease> <Symptom><Medical action word> <Age>

Examples:

heart & blood vessels disorders diagnosis tests
skin cancer treatment alternatives
urinary tract infections medication side effects
migraine headache pain prevention
coping with genitals herpes

Search Word Rotation

You focus on a particular *<Disease Word>* and then add *<Medical Action Words>* one search at a time. You work your way through the various types of knowledge needed to address issues you can encounter at the various stages of the disease or treatment.

You start at the beginning of the *<Medical Action Words>* and conduct one search after the other, reading and evaluating the results along the way, as you work though a short list of the action words.

First type in:

<Disease Word> and <Medical Action Words>

Then keep the first word the same but change the second word like this:

Search 1: *<Disease Word> <Causes>*
Search 2: *<Disease Word> <Identification>*
Search 3: *<Disease Word> <Diagnosis>*
Search 4: *<Disease Word> <Control>*
Search 5: *<Disease Word> <Treatment>*
Search 6: *<Disease Word> <Therapy>*
Search 7: *<Disease Word> <Medications>*

Search 8: *<Disease Word> <Side effects>*
Search 9: *<Disease Word> <Rehabilitation>*

Get the idea? You rotate through the different *<Medical Action Words>* one at a time. You learn about each subject from the web sites you find as you go through the cycle of medical actions. You start at disease identification and onset and work your way the life cycle of your disease through to treatment and rehabilitation.

Here are some examples:

<u>thyroid disease symptoms</u>
<u>thyroid disease causes</u>
<u>thyroid disease control</u>
<u>thyroid disease management</u>
<u>thyroid disease treatment alternatives</u>
<u>thyroid disease therapy</u>
<u>thyroid disease medications</u>
<u>thyroid disease medication side effects</u>

Phrase and Concept Searches

Turn a typical question or phrase into the actual words you use to search. The search string construction is like this:

<u><phrase> <disease></u>
<u>How to manage <disease></u>
<u>How to survive <condition></u>
<u>How do I survive <condition></u>

Examples:

<u>how do I survive anorexia?</u>
<u>learn how to survive my depression</u>
<u>how to survive a heart attack</u>
<u>preventing child abuse</u>
<u>living with an alcoholic</u>
<u>how do I deal with my allergies?</u>
<u>what should I do about my back pain?</u>
<u>Use the key information source words</u>

Search Various Sources of Information

To make sure you get valid medical health information, you should focus your searches on the high potential sources of quality medical and health information. To do this you can use the *<Information Source Words>* in your search string like this:

<Disease Words> <Information Source Word>

The *<Information Source Words>* include terms associated with the entire spectrum of government agencies, businesses, companies, corporations large and small, professional associations, nonprofit organizations, and universities, colleges, and other educational institutions.

For example:

medical health information professional associations
health information government
patient care information foundations

Use these one at a time and rotate through them. Use the *<Information Source words>* with the *<Disease Words>* to improve your general knowledge, identify specific treatment alternatives and actions, or improve your skills in dealing with medical information, doctors, and institutions.

You will find that many of the source organizations provide excellent educational search resources.

You can, of course, use the Minus Dot Com Trick to quickly eliminate the commercial web sites and separate the organizational sites government sites, and educational sites.

Use Location and Date Words

Use location and date words at the end of your search string.

<Disease Words> <Source Word> <Location Words> <Date Words>

For example:

<u>diabetes educators Los Angeles California 2002</u>
<u>breast cancer support groups Georgia 2002</u>

Use *<Location Words>* one at a time and rotate through them.

You can use *<Location Words>* with the *<Disease Words>* and *<Source Words>* to find ways to improve your general knowledge of facilities and health care providers or institutions in the areas nearby to where you live or need help.

CREATE A SEARCH STRING

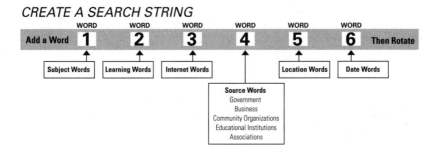

QUICKSTART
Go to www.Google.com.

CREATE A SEARCH STRING

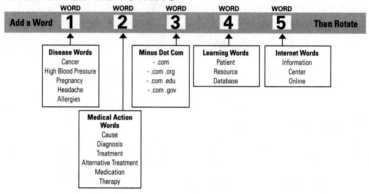

Then search on the words you selected. Study the results. Surf. Learn and enjoy what you find.

Then create another search string using different words and search again.

Create Your Own Search String to Research Any Question or Problem

Identify any subject that interests you. Make a list of key terms, scientific terminology, or related words.

Use these as your initial subject word. Then add appropriate Action Words, Learning Words, and Internet Words to create your search string.

five

Discovering the Fountain of Eternal Youth

This section of the book provides you with magic search words and recommended search strings for you to use to find the best information quickly on a wide range of commonly searched health topics.

Each area of medicine has it's own special terminology. The key words that uncover the best information are provided here for you to use.

Once you know what topic you are interested in, use the tactics and search strategies and techniques introduced in the first part of the book to find exactly what you are looking for.

Each specific topic starts with a short section that highlights the best search strings to use to get to the best information quickly. The key search string word groups are then presented along with the key magic search words associated with that word group. The short lists of *<Learning Words>* provided here are intended to get you started. Refer to the more detailed lists of *<Learning Words>* and *<Internet Words>* to conduct more effective searches.

Specific Medical & Health Topics

Topic	Page
Aging, Elder Care, Long-Term Care and Rehabilitation	63
Allergies, Asthma, & Immunology	64
Alternative Health & Medical Treatment	66
Blood, Circulatory & Lymphatic System	67
Bones, muscles, joints, orthopedics & physical therapy	68
Cancer	70
Chiropractic Care	72
Colds and the Flu	73
Death & Dying	74
Dental and Oral Care	75
Diabetes, Hormonal & other Immune System Disorders	77
Digestive System & Gastrointestinal Illness	78
Ears and Hearing	80
Eating, Foods and Nutrition	81
Emergencies, Poison Control & Safety	83
Eye Care & Vision	85
Family & Parenting	87
Fitness & Exercise	89
Foot Care	89
Heart Disease and Cardiology	90
Headache and Migraine	92
Infections	93
Lungs & Airways	94
Medication & Drugs	95
Men's Health	97
Mental Health & Psychiatry	98
Nervous System and Neurology	100
Physical & Developmental Disabilities	102
Plastic Surgery	102
Sex & Fertility	103
Sexual Disorders	105
Skin Care and Skin Diseases	106
Sleep Disorders	108
Social Problems, Physical, Sexual Problems	109
Sports Medicine and Injuries	110
Substance Abuse	111
Surgery	112
Tests, Tools and Calculators	113
Travel and Health	115
Women's Health	116
X-rays, Radiology and Nuclear Medicine	118

Aging, Elder Care, Long-Term Care and Rehabilitation

CREATE A SEARCH STRING

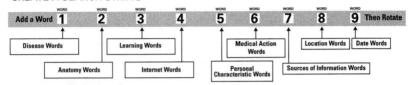

\<Medical Specialties\>
Gerontology   Genomic research   Geriatric research

\<Learning Words\>
Ask an expert aging   Ask a professional   A to Z
Ask a doctor elder care

\<Information Words\>
Aeveos   Aging body   Diseases of the elderly
Aging   Bodily changes   Implications of illness

\<Symptom Words\>
Disability   Pain   Skin diseases
Fatigue   Poor appetite   Sleeplessness
Gastrointestinal problems   Shortness of breath   Weight problems
Mental illness

\<Medical Issue Words\>
Diagnostic tools   Health well-being elderly   New therapies
Elder care   Increased longevity   Prolong vitality
Elderly rehabilitation   Long-term care   Senior health care
Gerontological society   Medication   information
Golden age

\<Location\>
Home health agencies   Physical therapy geriatrics   Resource centers *\<location\>*
    \<location\>   *\<location\>*
Nursing centers   Rehabilitation provider
    directory   directory

\<Facilities\>
Adult day care   Medical day care   Residential care facilities
Day hospitals   Mental Health day care   Retirement communities
Home care   Nursing Homes   Skilled nursing facilities
Hospice   Nutrition services   Social adult day care
Intermediate care facilities

\<Long-term Care\>

Adult day care elderly
Caregiver
Compare health care
   services
Compare health plans
Compare hospitals
Compare nursing homes
Cost of long-term care
Cost reimbursement

Effect on family
Eldercare facilities locator
Eldercare locator
Elders, seniors, matures,
   elderly, older persons
Free newsletter
Government sources
   information

Long-term nursing care
Network
Purchasing home medical
   equipment
Rehabilitation
Resource locators
Retirement and financial
   planning

\<Disease Words\>

Alzheimer's disease
Arthritis diagnosis
Bedsores
Cataracts
Dementia
Diabetes

Glaucoma
Heart attack
Hyperparathyroidism
Leukemia
Osteoporosis

Paget's disease
Parkinson's
Prostate cancer
Shingles
Stroke

\<Medical Action Words\>

Care
Early diagnosis
Family support
Medication

Medicine
Prognosis
Side effects
Signs

Support services
Symptoms
Therapy
Treatment

\<Phrase and Concept Words\>

Caring for an aging relative
Choosing a nursing home
Dealing with critical issues

Hiring home health care help
Involving the elderly in their
   own care

Making better health care
   choices

Allergies, Asthma, & Immunology

CREATE A SEARCH STRING

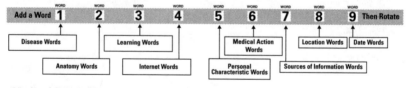

\<Medical Specialties\>

Allergists
Ear, Nose & Throat

Endocrinologists

Immunologists

\<Learning Words\>

A to Z
Ask the Doctor
Ask The Expert

Ask the Professional
Databases
Directories

FAQ's
Online consultants
Q&A's

\<Information Words\>

Allergic reaction
Antibodies

Antihistamines

Immune system

\<Causes\>

Air Pollution
Animals
Chemicals
Cosmetics
Drugs
Food

Grass
Irritants
Latex
Metals
Mold

Occupational allergies
   asthma
People
Plants
Spores
Triggers

\<Symptom Words\>

Anaphylactic shock
Coughing
Hives
Irritation pain
Itchy eyes

Nasal congestion
Raspy throat
Red eyes
Skin rashes

Sneezes
Sniffles
Stuffed Nose
Wheezing

\<Disease Words\>

Allergic Rhinitis
Anaphylaxis
Asthma
Cold

Dermatitis
Drug allergies
Food allergies
Hay fever

Insect allergies
Sinusitis
Urticaria
Welts

\<Medical Action Words\>

Alternatives
Avoidance
Diagnosis

Medications
Prevention
Reactions

Symptoms
Treatment

\<Medical Issue Words\>

Allergic reactions
Allergic to \<substance\>
   help
Allergies Genetics
Allergy intolerance
Allergy medicine overdose
Allergy sufferers
Allergy testing
Alternative health
Clinical studies
Controlling allergies
Controlling asthma
Effective treatment of
   \<symptom\>

Helpful hints for managing
   allergies \<type\>
Home Office Work
Homeopathy
Learning laboratory
Mold spores
Mold spore counts
   \<location\>
Mystery ailments food
   allergies
Participation studies
Pollen counts
Pollen counts \<location\>

Product alerts
Protecting against \<specific
   allergy\>
Protecting against allergies
Relief from \<symptom\>
Self-tests
Specialized diets
Teaching Patients about
   \<disease\>
Weather

<Medications>

Antihistamines	Home remedies	Non-prescription
Herbal remedies	Nasal Sprays	Prescription

Examples:

<u>ask the ear nose throat doctor online consultant</u>

<u>help sinus relief magazine articles</u>

<u>tips for managing hay fever</u>

<u>living with food allergies</u>

<u>allergies in the workplace</u>

Alternative Health & Medical Treatment

CREATE A SEARCH STRING

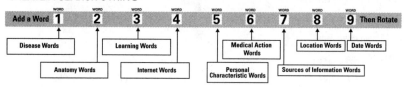

<Information Words>

Alternative medicine	Exercise therapy	Hypnosis
Aromatherapy	Fasting	Hypnotherapy
Auriculotherapy	Feldenkrais method	Interpersonal psychotherapy
Autogenic training	Flotation tanks	Ion generators
Ayurvedic medicine	Flower therapy	Journal writing
Behavior therapy	Gestalt therapy	Laetrile
Biofeedback	Ginseng	Leeches
Bodywork	Gravity immersion	Light therapy
Breathing techniques	Group therapy	Macrobiotics
Cell therapy	Heat therapy	Massage
Chinese herbs	Herbal medicine, forms,	Meditation
Chiropractic	types, medicinal value,	Music therapy
Cognitive therapy	indications,	Naturopathy
Complimentary medicine	contraindications, side	Nutritional therapy
Colon therapy	effects, controversy,	Oxygen therapy
Color therapy	abuse, poisoning, risks	Pet therapy
Computer therapy	Holistic medicine treatment,	Physiatry
Craniosacral	therapy, techniques,	Physiatrists
Detoxification	learning	Plant therapy
Dream analysis	Home remedies	Poetry therapy
Electro-convulsive therapy	Homeopathy	Polarity
Electrotherapy	Hydrotherapy	Progressive relaxation
Energy medicine	Hydrotherapy	Psychoanalysis

Reflexology
Rolfing
Self-help audiotapes
Stress management

Therapeutic touch
Time management
Touch therapy
Urine therapy

Vegetarian diet
Vision therapy
Yoga

Blood, Circulatory & Lymphatic System

CREATE A SEARCH STRING

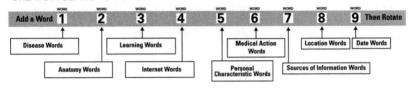

\<Medical Specialties\>

Hematology

\<Anatomy Words\>

Blood biology
Blood cells
Capillaries

Circulatory system
   \<Anatomy Words\>
Heart

Lymphatic system
   \<Anatomy Words\>
Spleen
Veins

\<Learning Words\>

A to Z
ABC's
Guides

Information resources
Manuals

Patient information
Patient resources

\<Disease Words\>

Abnormalities
Anemia
Bleeding disorders
Bleeding emergency
   treatment leukemia
Blood disorders

Diabetes
Hematology
Hemophiliac
Hodkin's disease
Immune system diseases
Leukemia

Lymphedema
Lymphomas
Plasma cell disorders
Red blood cell disorders
Sickle cell
White blood cell disorders

\<Medical Issue Words\>

Blood alcohol
Blood sample
Blood smear
Blood transfusion

Blood types
Bone marrow transplants
First aid
Plasma cell disorders

Poor clotting
Red blood cell disorders
Spleen disorders
White blood cell disorders

\<Medical Action Words\>

Alternatives
Diagnosis

Medication
Prevention

Resources
Treatment

<Symptom Words>

Bleeding from ears	Blood in stool	Blood pressure low
Bleeding from wounds	Blood in urine	Blood pressure normal
Blood in semen	Blood pressure high	

Examples:

Using Bandages

Using Tourniquets

Wound care guide

Wound care manual online

Wound cleaning

Effective wound care and cleaning

Wound care guide

Cleaning out a bad cut

What do I do if my semen has blood

Bones, muscles, joints, orthopedics & physical therapy

CREATE A SEARCH STRING

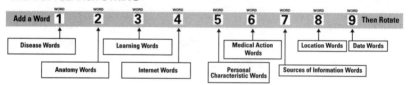

<Medical Specialties>

Chiropractics	Podiatry	Sports medicine
Orthopedics	Physical Therapy	

<Learning Words>

A to Z	Directory	Find an orthopedist
Ask a doctor	Disorders	Foot Ankle Information
Ask about *<subject word>*	FAQ's	Illnesses
Conditions	Find a therapist locator	Index

<Information Words>

Bone diseases	Foot problems	Paget's disease
Bone tumors	Musculoskeletal system	Physical Therapy
Chiropractic and bodywork professionals	Orthopedic Patient Information	Information
Exercise	Osteoarthritis	Podiatry Information
Fitness	Osteoporosis	Sports injuries

<Anatomy Words>

Ankle	Head	Ribs
Arms	Hip	Shoulders
Back	Knee	Skull
Cartilage	Leg	Spinal column
Elbow	Ligaments	Tendons
Foot	Muscles	Toes
Hands	Neck	Wrists

<Disease Words>

Achilles tendonitis	Dislocation	Repetitive strain injury
Ankle sprain	Fractures	Rheumatoid arthritis
Arch sprain	Gout	Runner's knee
Arthritis	Hammertoes	Scoliosis
Back sprains	Hernia	Shin splints
Baseball finger	Herniated disks	Sports injuries
Bone infections	Infections	Sports medicine injuries
Bone transplants	Joint replacement	Spurs
Bone tumors	Little leaguer's elbow	Stress fractures
Bunions	Muscle cramps	Tendonitis
Bursitis	Osteoporosis	Tennis elbow
Connective tissue disorders	Paget's Disease	Trauma
Degenerative disease	Poor posture	Unstable vertebrae
disorders	Pulled hamstrings	Weight lifter's back

<Symptom Words>

Aching	Fractures	Strains
Back Pain	Injured	Swelling
Bleeding	Painful joints	Swollen
Bone pain	Serious injury	Tenderness
Broken	Sore	Torn
Discoloration	Sprains	

<Medical Action Words>

Alternatives	Pain prevention	Proper posture
Diagnosis	Pain relief	Treatment
Fracture repair	Posture realignment	X-ray

<Medical Issue Words>

Athletic injuries	Consulting with a doctor	Patient-doctor relationship
Bone narrow transplant	Ergonomic resources	Supporting role of family
Chiropractors	Metabolic bone diseases	Types of arthritis
Choosing the right doctor		

Examples:

bones muscles joints diseases diagnosis
bones muscles joints diseases treatment
medical massage physical therapy
medical massage online illustrated guide
knee injury painful treatment
aching back pain therapy
slipped disk diagnosis treatment
sprained ankle hot cold therapy
hand wrist pain repetitive motion disorder
carpal tunnel syndrome treatment
torn ligament tendons leg pain management
children fractured arms diagnosis treatment
guide for the care of your back

Cancer

CREATE A SEARCH STRING

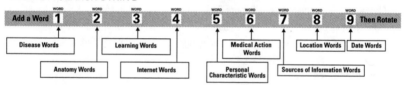

<Medical Specialties>
Oncology

<Learning Words>

A to Z	Ask About *<disease>*	Cancer treatment
An introduction to	Cancer information	information
<type of cancer>	resources	Information on Cancer

<Symptom Words>

Bleeding	Leaking	Pain
Growth changes in warts or	Lumps	Swelling
moles	Nagging cough or	Thickening
Inflammation	hoarseness	

<Medical Issue Words>

Avoiding cancer quackery	Causes of cancer	Cancer epidemiology
Bone marrow transplants	Cancer emergencies	Children with cancer

Hair lost prevention
Immunotherapy
Living with cancer

Patient care
Specialized cancer centers

Warning signs
Where to go

<Disease Words>

Bone cancer
Brain cancer
Breast cancer
Cervical cancer
Colon cancer
Connective tissue
Eye
Gastric

Hodgkin's disease
Intestinal cancer
Leukemia
Liver cancer
Lung Cancer
Lymphomas
Mouth, pharynx, larynx,
    throat

Multiple myeloma
Ovarian
Rectal cancer
Skin
Thyroid
Urinary tract
Uterine

<Medical Action Words>

Alternative therapies
Alternative therapies not
    approved
Causes
Chemotherapy
Clinical trials
Complications

Detection
Diagnosis
Emergencies
New approved treatments
Radiation therapy
Rehabilitation
Risk factors

Screening
Side effects
Staging
Surgery
Therapy
Treatment
Warning signs

Examples:

cancer symptoms identification

living with cancer

ask about cancer

cancer information for patients

cancer resources for Parkinson's disease

everything you wanted to know about bone marrow transplants

cancer care online assistance

surviving cancer

"100 types of cancer"

Chiropractic Care

CREATE A SEARCH STRING

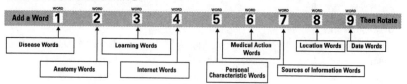

\<Medical Specialties\>

Chiropractics   Chiropractors

\<Learning Words\>

Associations	Organizations	Research information
Educational information	Professional	

\<Medical Issue Words\>

Alternative health	Homeopathic	Philosophy
Holism	Homeostasis	Regulatory role

\<Anatomy Words\>

Nervous system	Neuro-musculoskeletal system	Somatovisceraleffects
		Subluxation

\<Disease Words\>

Allergies	Digestive	Hearing impairment
Asthma	Energy improvement	Lethargy
Atitis media	Equilibrium	Lowered resistance
Back pain	Extremities	Pelvic
Bedwetting	Head and neck pain	Respiratory
Cardiac	Headache	Tonsillitis
Colic	Hearing	Vision

\<Medical Action Words\>

Acupuncture	Alternative health	Treatment
Adjustment	Diagnosis	Therapy
Alternative treatment		

Colds and the Flu

CREATE A SEARCH STRING

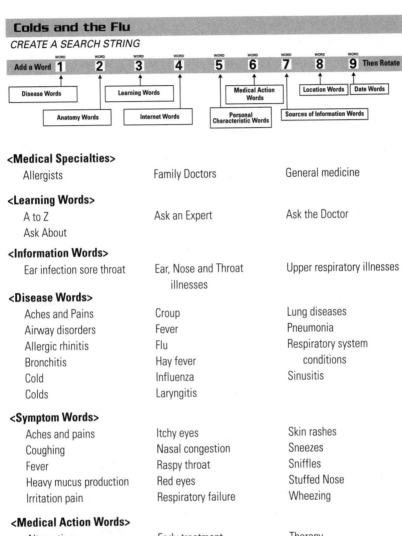

<Medical Specialties>

Allergists	Family Doctors	General medicine

<Learning Words>

A to Z	Ask an Expert	Ask the Doctor
Ask About		

<Information Words>

Ear infection sore throat	Ear, Nose and Throat illnesses	Upper respiratory illnesses

<Disease Words>

Aches and Pains	Croup	Lung diseases
Airway disorders	Fever	Pneumonia
Allergic rhinitis	Flu	Respiratory system
Bronchitis	Hay fever	conditions
Cold	Influenza	Sinusitis
Colds	Laryngitis	

<Symptom Words>

Aches and pains	Itchy eyes	Skin rashes
Coughing	Nasal congestion	Sneezes
Fever	Raspy throat	Sniffles
Heavy mucus production	Red eyes	Stuffed Nose
Irritation pain	Respiratory failure	Wheezing

<Medical Action Words>

Alternatives	Early treatment	Therapy
Diagnosis	Prevention	Treatment
Early diagnosis	Tests	

Examples:

treating a cold

getting a flu shot

which medication is best for a sore throat

home remedies for the flu

Death & Dying

CREATE A SEARCH STRING

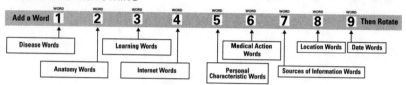

<Medical Specialties>

Forensic science	Gerontology	Pathology
Geriatrics		

<Learning Words>

A to Z	Government	Resources
Family Information	Patient Information	

<Information Words>

Advanced directives	Hospice care	Respite care
Causes of death	Legal preparations	Symptoms during fatal
Coming to terms	Living wills	illness
Durable power of attorney	Making choices	Time of dying
Effects on family	Nursing home care	Trusts, wills and estates
Home care	Predicting death	When death is near

<Causes>

Cancer	Leading	Smoking
Drugs	Mortality morbidity weekly	
Heart disease	report CDC	

<Medical Issue Words>

Advanced directions	Euthanasia	Nursing care
Aging	Evaluating care options	Nursing home care
Bereavement	Family care	Parents
<Caregivers> types	Family Support	Patient self-determination
Children	Grief support	Paying for care
Choices available	Grieving Process	Planning for death and
Comparing types of care	Hospice care	dying
Death of a loved one	Hospital care	Respite Care
Durable power of attorney	Human mortality	Selecting care
Dying process	Living wills	Suicide, legal issues, view
Dying with dignity	Locating care facilities	and practices of doctors
Effects on *<family>*	Natural death	Widows
Emotional support		

<Medical Action Words>

Alternatives	Identification	Prediction
Assessment	Managing	Recovery
Coping with	Medication	Rehabilitation
Dealing with	Pain management	Risk of Dying *<disease>*
End-of-life issues	Planning	Treatment

Examples:

discussing death with children
coping with a loved ones death
helping someone through grief
surviving the death of your loved one
family survival guide

Dental and Oral Care

CREATE A SEARCH STRING

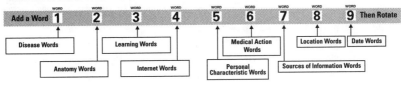

<Medical Specialties>

Dentistry	Oral care	Periodontics
Endontists	Oral health	Prostodontics
Orthodontics	Pedodontics	

<Learning Words>

A to Z	Ask an Expert	Guides
Ask About	Ask the Doctor	Manuals

<Information Words>

Dentists language	Dental terminology	Periodontal diseases
Dental terms	Dental anatomy	

<Anatomy Words>

Bonding	Gums	Root canal
Bridges	Lower Jaw	Teeth
Crowns	Mouth	Upper Jaw
Filings		

<Medical Issue Words>

Cleaning your teeth
Dental patient education
    information
Dental visits

Emergency treatment
Locating a dentist
Oral hygiene

Preventing tooth decay
Selecting a dentist
Visiting the dentist

<Disease Words>

Abnormal jaw
Abscesses
Baby teeth
Bad breath
Burned tongue and palate
Cancer
Canker sores
Caries
Cavities
Chewing tobacco
Cleft lip
Cleft palate
Color changes
Cold sores
Cracked teeth
Dental caries
Dental problems
Discoloration teeth
Dry mouth
Face and mouth injuries

Fluoride
Fractured jaw
Fractured teeth
Gingivitis
Growths
Gum diseases (periodontal)
Halitosis
Impacted teeth
Infections
Jaw fracture
Jaw pain
Knocked out teeth
Lip biting
Lip problems
Lock Jaw
Loose teeth
Malformed teeth
Missing teeth
Mouth odor
Mouth sores

Oral cancer
Oral herpes
Pain
Periodontal disease
Pulling teeth
Saliva diseases
Salivary gland problems
Smoking
Taste disorders
Teeth *<Disease Words>*
Toothaches
Tooth decay
Tooth disorders
Toothpaste
Traumatic injury *<action word>*
Trench mouth
X-rays

<Medical Action Words>

Alternatives
Dental checkups
Diagnosis

Identification
Physical Therapy
Prevention

Symptoms
Treatment

Examples:

best way to whiten your teeth
preventing child mouth injuries sports
preventing tooth decay
getting rid of bad breath
how to stop biting lips
selecting a dentist

Diabetes, Hormonal & other Immune System Disorders

CREATE A SEARCH STRING

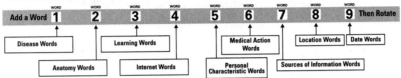

<Medical Specialties>

Endocrinology   Internal Medicine   Immune system disorders
Immunology

<Learning Words>

A to Z   Ask an Expert   Ask the Doctor
Ask About

<Anatomy Words>

Adrenal gland   Immune system physiology   Pituitary gland
Antibodies   Lymph glands   Primary immune deficiency
Endocrine system   Lymphatic system   Thyroid gland
Immune system anatomy

<Disease Words>

Acquired immunodeficiency   Diabetes mellitus   Hypothyoidism
    disorders   Goiter   Immunodeficiency disorders
Adrenal gland disorders   Grave's Disease   Low blood sugar
Allergic reactions   Hives   Pituitary gland disorders
Anaphylaxis   Hyperthyroidism   Thyroid cancer
Carcinoid   Hypoglycemia   Thyroid gland disorders

<Medical Action Words>

Alternatives   Emergency care   Symptoms
Causes   Identification   Treatment
Common misconceptions   Medication   Warning signs
Complications   Signs of

<Medical Issue Words>

Abnormalities   Diabetes mellitus   Hyperglycemia
Adolescence   Diet   Hypoglycemia
Childhood   Education centers   Juvenile diabetes
Complications   Emergency care   Patient information
Diabetes   Elderly   Pregnancy
Diabetes in children   Foot care   Smoking

Examples:

<u>help for parents of children with primary immune deficiency</u>
<u>managing your diabetes</u>
<u>diabetes recipes cookbooks</u>
<u>diabetes interactive tests</u>
<u>diabetes articles fact sheets</u>

Digestive System & Gastrointestinal Illness

CREATE A SEARCH STRING

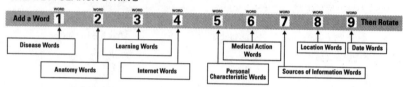

\<Medical Specialties>
Gastroenterology   Internal Medicine

\<Learning Words>
A to Z   Ask an expert   Diagnostic center
Alphabetical index   Find a doctor   Patient information
Ask a doctor   GI Physician locator

\<Information Words>
Digestive system   Gastrointestinal online   Gastrointestinal system
                                 layperson

\<Anatomy Words>
Digestive system anatomy   Intestines   Pancreas
Digestive system diagrams   Kidney   Small Intestine
   pictures animations   Large Intestine   Stomach
Esophagus   Liver   Upper GI
Gallbladder   Lower GI

\<Disease Words>
Abscesses   Botulism   Constipation
Abdominal illnesses   Bowel movement disorders   Crohn's Disease
Acid reflux   Cancers   Diarrhea
Anal fissures   Chemical food poisoning   Digestive diseases
Anal itching   Cholera   information
Anal polyps   Cirrhosis of the liver   Digestive disorders
Backpacker's disease   Colitis   Diverticular diseases
Bleeding   Congenital defects   End-stage renal disease

Esophagus
Fecal incontinence
Food poisoning
Foreign objects swallowed
Gallbladder disease
Gallstones
Gastritis
Gastrointestinal bleeding
Gastrointestinal diseases
Gastrointestinal pain
Gastrointestinal problems
Gastrointestinal ulcers
Giardia
Growths of the intestines

Halitosis
Heartburn
Hemorrhoids
Hepatitis
Hernia
Incontinence
Indigestion
Intestinal cancer
Intestinal diseases
Intestinal gas
Jaundice
Kidney disease
Kidney stones

Lactose intolerance
Liver disease or disorders
Malabsorption
Pancreas
Peptic ulcers
Peritonitis
Renal failure
Rotavirus
Stomach disorders
Traveler's Diarrhea
Ulcers
Urinary incontinence
Urinary tract infections

<Symptom Words>

Abdominal gas
Bleeding
Bloating
Blockage
Constipation

Diarrhea
Difficulty swallowing
Farting
Inflamation
Intestinal gas

Nausea
Pain
Ulcers
Vomiting

<Medical Issue Words>

Abdominal pain self care
Abdominal pain self tests
Corrosive substances
    injestion

Cookbooks *<disease>*
Food and eating
Malnutrition

Nutrition
Overweight

<Medical Action Words>

Alternatives
Complications
Diagnosis

Diagnostic tests
Prevention
Symptoms

Therapy
Treatment

Examples:

how your digestive system works

facts and fallacies

treating dehydration in a child

gallstones pain diagnosis treatment

getting rid of severe heartburn

Ears and Hearing

CREATE A SEARCH STRING

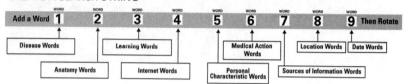

\<Medical Specialties\>
Audiology   Audiometrics

\<Learning Words\>
ABC's	Directories	Guides
A to Z	Databases	Manuals

\<Information Words\>
Audiology patient information resources	Ears and hearing diseases	Hearing aids
Ears and hearing disorders	Hearing education awareness	Patient information

\<Anatomy Words\>
Acoustic nerve	Cochlea	Stirrup
Anvil	Hammer	Tympanic membrane
Auricle	Outer ear	

\<Disease Words\>
Age-related hearing loss	Foreign bodies	Punctured eardrum
Blockages	Growths	Ringing in ears
Ear wax	Hearing loss	Sudden deafness
Cysts	Hearing test	Swimmer's ear
Deafness	Inner ear disorders	Tinitis
Earache	Occupational hearing loss	Tumors
Ear disorders	Outer ear disorders	Vestibular disorders
Eardrum injuries	Sinus disorders	

\<Symptom Words\>
Balance	Ear blockage	Ear infection
Dizziness	Ear buzzing	Ear injury
Ear ache	Ear unclogging altitude	Ear lobe injury
Ear bleeding		

\<Medical Action Words\>
Alternatives	Identification	Prevention
Diagnosis	Medication	Treatment

Examples:

why do my ears ring

ear infection treatment

sudden hearing loss causes treatment

something is stuck in my child's ear

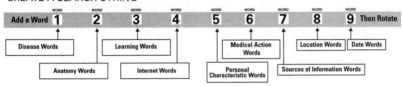

Eating, Foods and Nutrition

CREATE A SEARCH STRING

<Learning Words>

Ask a Dietitian	Dictionary of *<nutritional*	Guides
Ask an Expert *<type>*	*terms>*	Manuals
<disease> <illness>	Glossary of culinary terms	

<Information Words>

Carbohydrates	Malnutrition	Salt balance
Diet	Micronutrients	Starvation
Fats	Minerals	Vitamins
Food	Nutrition	Water
Importance of *<Medical*	Protein	Water balance
issue>	Salt	Weight control
Macronutrients		

<Medical Issue Words>

Anemia	Eating fruits and vegetables	Public health nutrition
Cooking utensils, hygiene,	Excess	School nutrition
cooking tips,	Healthy eating, recipes, diet	Sodium
Deficiencies	Patient nutrition	Taking care of *<problem>*
Eating fit, healthy eating,		

<Disease Words>

Acid-base imbalance	Low magnesium	*<Specific vitamin>*
Acidosis	Low phosphate	deficiency
Alkalosis	Low potassium	*<Specific vitamin>* excess
Cholesterol	Malnutrition	*<Specific mineral>*
Dehydration	Obesity	deficiency
High sodium	Salt imbalance	*<Specific mineral>* excess
Low calcium		Starvation

<Symptom Words>

Nausea	Pain	Urinary Tract Infections
Overweight	Tired	

<Special topics>

Diabetes, diabetics, recipes, dining, healthy living

Family health, nutrition

Herbs, medicinal properties, types of, dangers of

Important facts, food sources, functions in the body, interactions, recommended usage, symptoms, toxicity, deficiency, safety information

Low fat, low calorie, how low can you go, fat-free

Minerals, types of: calcium, magnesium, iron, potassium, phosphorus, zinc, copper, manganese

Proteins, amino acids,

Recipes, salads, vegetables

Vegetarians, vegans

Vitamins, types of: A, C, thiamin, riboflavin, niacin, B6, B12

<Food Types>

Appetizers	Nutrition analysis tools & calculators	Soups
Health food substitutions		Substitutes
Meat	Nutritional analysis	Sugars, sweets, candy
Milk, dairy products	*<specific food>*	Supplements
Non-dairy, dairy free	Pasta	Training nutrition
	Salads	Vegetables

<Food Issues>

Bad bugs	Food buying, preparation, storage	Foods (eggs, vegetables, meats, sugars, fats, breads, etc.)
Drinks		
Epicurean, Epicurious,	Food contamination control prevention	
Food and drug interactions		Junk food, fast food, facts, myths
Food borne natural toxins basic facts	Food poisoning	nutrition drinks
	Food pyramid	
Food borne pathogenic organisms handbook	Food safety, food borne illnesses	

<Phrase and Concept Words>

Biggest Mistakes bodybuilders Nutrition	Impress your date *<nutritional terms>*

Emergencies, Poison Control & Safety

CREATE A SEARCH STRING

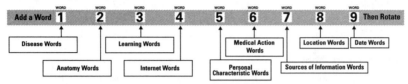

<Medical Specialties>

Emergency medicine	Occupational Health
Industrial Health	Paramedics

<Learning Words>

A to Z	First aid educational	Medic alert
Accidents	information	Medical emergencies
Ambulance	First aid educational	Medical health hotlines
Disaster	information	Medical health hotlines toll-
Disaster Plan	First aid treatment for	free
Disaster Plan Checklist	*<disorder>*	Mental health hotlines
Emergency aid	First aid treatment for	Online emergency medical
Emergency first steps	*<injury>*	management database
Emergency medical	First aid supplies checklist	Online emergency medical
attention	First responder emergency	management guide
Emergency medicine	response manual	Online first aid manual
Emergency medical	Hospital emergency	Poison control center *<Your*
technicians (EMT's)	*<nearest City, State>*	*State>*
First aid	Hospital emergency room	Quick guide first aid
First aid by emergency	*<Name hospital>*	Victim or patient
paramedics	Hospital emergency rooms	transportation

<Safety Precautions>

At home	Entrance	Medicine Cabinet
Automobile	Farm/Country	Motorcycle
Basement/Utility	Fire prevention	Road/Highway
Rooms/Workroom	Garden/Garage/Backyard	Snow skiing
Bathroom	Hiking	Stairs
Bedroom	Jet ski	Water
Bicycle	Kitchen	Water skiing
Boat	Living Room, Den, Family	Winter
Camping	Room	Workplace

<Medical Action Words>

Accident prevention	CPR infants	CPR adults
Causes	CPR children	Diagnosis

Emergency diagnosis
Equipment
Evaluation
Search and rescue
Home remedy

Home treatment
Life support
Prevention
Preventing
Rescue

Supplies
Symptoms
Triage
Treatment
Warning signs

<Medical Issue Words>

Airway obstruction
Altitude sickness
Amputations
Anaphylactic shock
Asphyxia
Biological materials
Biological warfare
Bites and stings
Bleeding
Breathing difficulty
Broken Bones
Bruises
Burns
Burns, major
Burns, minor
Carbon monoxide
Cardiac arrest
Cardiopulmonary
   resuscitation (CPR)
Chemical burns
Chemicals injected
Chemical ingested
Chest pain
Choking
Concussion
Convulsions
Coughing up blood
Dealing with *<situation>*
Dehydration
Dental emergencies
Diabetic coma/insulin shock
Drowning
Drug complications
Drug overdose
Drug withdrawal
Ear, foreign material in

Electrical burns
Electrical injury
Electrocution
Emergency childbirth
Emergency hospitalization
Epilepsy
Eye, foreign matter in
Eye injuries
Fainting
Fever
Food poisoning
Foreign bodies, ear, eye,
   skin
Fracture
Frostbite
Gangrene
Handling hurt people
Hazardous materials
Hazardous waste
Head injury
Head, neck and back
   injuries
Heart attack
Heat cramps
Heat exhaustion
Heat stroke
Heimlich maneuver
Hemorrhage
Herbal medicines
Hypothermia
Industrial accidents
Industrial poisons
Insect stings
Injuries
Internal injuries

Loss of consciousness
Managing *<situation>*
Material safety data sheets
   (MSDS)
Nosebleed
Obstructed breathing
Overexposure
Poisons
Poisonous plants
Poisonous substances
Poisoning
Poison Ivy, Oak and Sumac
Poisonous plants
Protecting against *<threat*
   of specific harm>
Radiological accidents
Radiation
Rape
Seizure
Septic shock
Severe cuts
Shock
Snakebites
Sprains
Stings
Strains
Stroke
Suffocation
Sunburn
Sun and heat
Toxic Substances
Unconscious
Vomiting
Vomiting blood
Whiplash

<Phrase and Concept Words>

Dealing with a medical   Managing a shock victim
   emergency   What to do

Examples:

first aid educational information
what to do in a burn emergency
wilderness emergency first aid
children severe cut bleeding treatment
first aid treatment for shock
<Specific Poison> diagnosis treatment
<Specific Poison> handling storage first aid

Eye Care & Vision

CREATE A SEARCH STRING

Add a Word	WORD 1	WORD 2	WORD 3	WORD 4	WORD 5	WORD 6	WORD 7	WORD 8	WORD 9 Then Rotate

Disease Words	Learning Words		Medical Action Words	Location Words	Date Words

Anatomy Words	Internet Words	Personal Characteristic Words	Sources of Information Words

<Medical Specialties>

Cataract and Refractive   Ophthalmology
   surgery   Optometry

<Learning Words>

A to Z   Database   Manuals
All about   Directories   Safety
Ask an Expert   Guides

<Anatomy Words>

Cornea   Optic nerve   Tear Ducts
Iris   Retina   Tear glands
Lens   Sclera   Vitreous humor

<Medical Issue Words>

Bruises   Cuts   Eye doctors
Chemical burns   Eclipses   Eye examinations
Color vision   Eye *<disease>* index   Eye glass lenses
Common Eye Diseases   Eye anatomy   Eye glasses
Computer vision problems   Eye Care Aids   Foreign bodies
Contact lenses   Eye care information   Low vision

Ophthalmology Patient
    Information
Optometry Information
    Resources
Safety

Solar burns
Sports and eye protection
Sun glasses
Sunburn

Vision
Vision conditions
Vision problems
Vision testing

<Disease Words>

Allergies
Astigmatism
Blindness
Bruises
Cataracts
Chemical burns
Color blindness
Conjunctivitis (Pink eye)
Corneal disorders
Crossed eyes

Cuts
Drooping eyelids
Eye injuries
Eye socket injuries
Eye lid disorders
Farsightedness
Foreign bodies
Glaucoma
High blood pressure
Impact injuries

Light sensitivity
Loss of vision diseases
Macular degeneration
Nearsightedness
Optic nerve disorders
Retinal detachment
Retinal disorders
Styes in the eye
Tear gland disorders
Usher's syndrome

<Medical Action Words>

Alternatives
Diagnosis

Treatment
Prevention

Protection
Safety

<Symptom Words>

Blind spots
Double vision
Hemorrhage

Jerking eyes
Protruding eyes

Rolling eyes
Spots

<Phrase and Concept Words>

Dealing with an eye injury

Preventing sports eye
    injuries

Removing a hair from your
    eye

Examples:

<u>current news about age-related macular degeneration</u>
<u>why should I get an eye examination</u>
<u>sports and eye protection injury prevention</u>
<u>how to treat conjunctivitis</u>
<u>selecting the right prescription sunglasses</u>
<u>buying contact lenses</u>

Family & Parenting

CREATE A SEARCH STRING

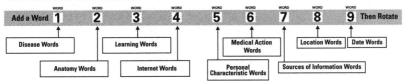

<Medical Specialties>

Pediatrics	Psychology
Psychiatry	Obstetrics/Gynocology

<Learning Words>

<age> <disease> <action word>	Ask the doctor	Health child care A to Z
Ask a professional	Family doctor	Online handbook
Ask an expert	Family physician	Safe child care ABC's

<Family Words>

Christian Parenting	Married Parents	Parent to parent
Dad to dad	Mom to mom	Single Parents

<Childhood Diseases>

Appendicitis	Head lice	Reye's syndrome
Asthma	Infancy	Rubella
Chickenpox	Influenza	Scarlet fever
Childhood	Kawasaki's disease	School years
Colds	Measles	Sore throat
Convulsions	Mumps	Tonsillitis
Ear infections	Preschool	Whooping cough
First year	Psychoses	Worms

<Adolescence>

Intellectual changes	Psychological changes	Teenagers
Moral development	Sexuality	Teens
Physical development		

<Parenting>

Aging Parents	Eating	Parenting *<specific subject>*
Being a parent	Eating disorders	*<age>*
Choosing a Physician	Home schooling	Parents of multiples
Dealing with difficult children	Managing Television	Playing
Discipline	Medical Health Hotlines Toll-Free	Schooling
Driving		Traveling

<Medical Issue Words>

Acne

Anorexia nervosa

Asthma

Attention Deficit Disorder
    ADD/ADHD

Battered child syndrome

Bulimia

Cancer

Child abuse

Child birth

Child death

Chronic inflammatory bowel
    disease

Contraception

Depression

Diabetes

Disabilities

Dyslexia

Epilepsy

Fitness exercise

Handicaps

Hearing loss

Hearing loss

Hepatitis

Immunizations

Incest

Iron-deficiency anemia

Lice, head lice, scabies

Masturbation

Migraine headache

Mononucleosis

Obesity

Out of control behavior

Poison

Rape

Scholl problems

Scoliosis

Seizures

Sexual fantasies

Sleep

Sports injuries

Suicide

Thyroid problems

Tuberculosis

Urinary tract infections

Venereal disease

Vision

Vision and eye care, glasses

Weight

<Phrase and Concept Words>

Advice for parents
    <condition>

Caring for child *<disease>*

Child's medicine cabinet
    safety

Cool stuff for *<age> <health>*

Cool stuff for *<age> <safety>*

Coping with tragedy

Dealing with Stigma from
    mentally ill relative

Managing child *<illness>*

My visit to the
    <medical facility>

My visit to the Dentist

My visit to the Doctor

My visit to the Hospital

Sibling support *<illness>*

Taking care of a sick child

Tips for living with

Examples:

<u>infant potty training bedwetting</u>

<u>teenagers discipline challenges of not hitting</u>

<u>reading to children</u>

<u>parenting your teens bedroom</u>

<u>Keeping your child out of harm's way</u>

Fitness & Exercise

CREATE A SEARCH STRING

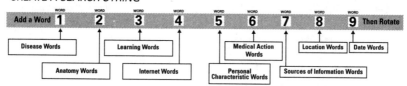

<Information Words>

Aerobics	Exercise programs	Swimming
Avoiding injuries	Meditation	Video exercise
Bicycling	Muscle builders	Walking
Body builders	Muscle tone	Warming up
Burning fat	Obesity	Weight loss
Cardiovascular exercise	Overweight	Weight management
Cooling down	Preventing injuries	Weightlifting
Cross country skiing	Sports bodies	Workout
Dancing	Stretching	Yoga
Exercise fundamentals		

<Phrase and Concept Words>

Biggest Mistakes athletes make	Help yourself to better fitness	Ten Great Tips to better fitness
Choosing the right exercise	Starting an exercise program	

Examples:

dangers of not exercising

how exercise benefits health

health problems overweight

Foot Care

CREATE A SEARCH STRING

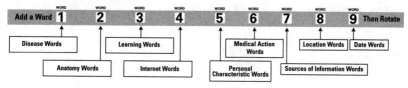

<Medical Specialty>

Podiatry

<Learning Words>

A to Z	Patient Information	Resources
Ask a doctor		

<Information Words>

Ankle problems
Common athletic foot
   injuries
Common athletic foot
   problems
Common foot problems

Foot afflictions
Foot ailments
Foot anatomy
Foot conditions
Foot deformities
Foot information

Podiatric patient
   information
Podiatry
Podiatry online
Podiatry quick reference

<Anatomy Words>

Ankle
Feet

Foot
Heel

Phalanges
Toes

<Medical Issue Words>

Achilles tendonitis
Aging feet
Amputation
Bunions
Corns

Diabetes
Fibromyalgia
Flat feet
Foot oder
Foot surgery

Hammertoe
Heel spurs
Ingrown toenails
Shin splints
Stress fractures

<Medical Action Words>

Alternatives
Diagnosis *<disorders>*

Foot-related *<products>*
Symptoms

Treatment *<disorders>*

<Phrase and Concept Words>

Fighting foot fungus

Healthy toenails

Managing a broken foot

Examples:

<u>diabetic foot risk calculator</u>
<u>sports-related foot injuries</u>
<u>air shoes for aerobics</u>
<u>top ten foot problems</u>

Heart Disease and Cardiology

CREATE A SEARCH STRING

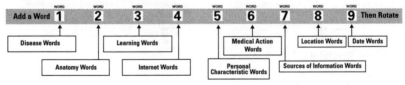

<Medical Specialties>

Cardiology

Cardiovascular medicine

\<Learning Words\>

A to Z   Patient Information   Resources
Ask a doctor

\<Information Words\>

Healthy heart guide   Heart Conditions   Heart surgery online
Heart & Circulatory   Identification Diagnosis   consumer resource
   problems   Treatment   Online interactive tools
Heart & Stroke   Heart Online exploration   heart
Heart Disease Index   Heart surgery online patient   Online interactive
Heart Disorders Index   information   cardiology tools

\<Medical Issue Words\>

Abnormal heart rhythms   Coronary artery disease   Hypertension
Aneurisms   Coronary heart disease   Lack of exercise
Angina   Diet   Lifestyle
Angioplasty   Drinking   Low blood pressure
Artheriosclerosis   Exercise   Medication
Bypass surgery   Heart attack   Obesity
Cardiac arrhythmias   Heart disease   Risk factors
Cardiovascular disease   Heart failure   Shock
Cholesterol   Heart tumors   Smoking
Congenital heart defects   Heart valve disorders   Sudden cardiac death
Congestive heart failure   High blood pressure   Surgery

\<Medical Action Words\>

Diagnosis   Exercise tolerance testing   Treatment
Identification   Prognosis   Therapy
Emergency   Tests   Surgery

\<Phrase and Concept Words\>

Managing after a heart   Preventing heart disease   What to do if you have
   attack   Treating heart pain   heart disease

Examples:

prevention of stroke

recovering after a stroke

tips for preventing a heart attack

calculating heart attack survival

evaluating chest pain

heart disease in women

living with heart disease

Headache and Migraine

CREATE A SEARCH STRING

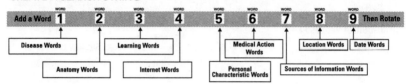

<Learning Words>

A to Z	Information Centers	Resources
Q & A	Physician Referrals	Resource Centers
Information		

<Information Words>

Cluster headaches	Hypertension	Sleeplessness
Glaucoma	Migraine	Tension headaches
Headaches	Sinus problems	Vertigo

<Symptom Words>

Chronic Head Pain	Lethargy	Stress
Depression	Migraine	Suffering
Headache	Pain	Tension
Jitteriness		

<Medical Action Words>

Advice	Education	Medication
Alternatives	Treatment	Prevention
Diagnosis	Management	

<Headache Types>

Analgesic-abuse	Post-traumatic	Tension
Cluster	Sinus	Throbbing

<Phrase and Concept Words>

Coping with migraine	Dealing with severe headaches

Examples:

how to better manage headache pain

coping with a migraine

self-diagnosis tool for migraine

I've got an Excedrin headache

migraine and children

Infections

CREATE A SEARCH STRING

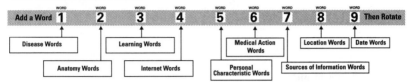

<Medical Specialties>
Internal medicine

<Learning Words>

A to Z	All about	Ask an expert
Ask about	Ask a doctor	Databases

<Biology Words>

Bacteria, bacterium	Lymph	Parasites
Blood	Microorganisms	Skin
Ear	Muscle	Symbiotes
Fungi, Fungus	Nose Throat	Virus, Viruses
Lungs		

<Information Words>

Blood changes	Cell changes	Effect on human body
Body defenses against infection	Defense mechanisms	Organ changes

<Medical Issue Words>

Drugs	Medication	Vaccinations
Fever	Sexually transmitted diseases	
Immunizations		

<Disease Words>

Abscesses	Herpes	Parasitic infections
AIDS	HIV	Plague
Candida	Hookworms	Rabies
Cat-scratch	Influenza	Respiratory infections
Cholera	Leprosy	Retrovirus
Common cold	Leprosy	Ricketts
Fungal infections	Lyme disease	Rubella
Gangrene	Malaria	Salmonella
Giardiasis	Measles	Scarlet Fever
Gonorrhea	Meningitis	Shingles
Hantavirus	Mononucleosis	Spirochetes
Hepatitis B	Mumps	Staph infections

Syphyllis	Toxic shock syndrome	Tuberculosis
Tapeworms	Trichinosis	Typhoid fever
Tetanus	Tuberculosis	Viral infections

<Symptoms>

Bleeding	Headache	Redness
Fever	Pain	Swelling

<Medical Action Words>

Alternatives	Identification	Side Effects
Assessment	Prevention	Symptoms
Diagnosis	Risk factors	Treatment

<Phrase and Concept Words>

Avoiding syphyllis	Dealing with infection	Managing infections

Lungs & Airways

CREATE A SEARCH STRING

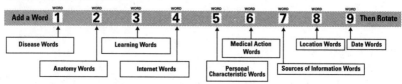

<Medical Specialties>
Internal medicine

<Learning Words

A to Z	Ask a doctor	Directory
Ask an expert	Database	

<Information Words>

Allergies	Control of breathing	Occupational lung disease
Asbestos	Gas exposure	Respiration
Beryllium	Lung diseases	Respiratory function
Chemical exposure	Lung disorders	Smoking

<Anatomy Words>

Alveolus	Epiglottis	Pharynx
Bronchiole	Larynx	Trachea
Bronchus	Lungs	

<Disease Words>

Asthma	Asbestosis	Bronchitis
Acute respiratory stress	Berylliosis	Chronic obstructive
Allergic diseases	Black lung	pulmonary disease

Cystic fibrosis	Pleurisy	Pulmonary embolism
Legionnaire's disease	Obstructive airway diseases	Pulmonary fibrosis
Lung abscess	Occupational lung disease	Strep throat
Lung cancer	Pneumonia	

<Symptom Words>

Blue discoloration	Hoarse	Throat pain
Chest pain	Raspy throat	Wheezing
Cough	Shortness of breath	

<Medical Action Words>

Alternatives	Medication	Symptoms
Diagnosis	Prevention	Therapy
Diagnostic Testing	Prognosis	Treatment

Medication & Drugs

CREATE A SEARCH STRING

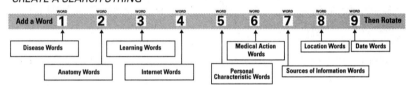

<Medical Specialties>

| Clinical Pharmacology | Pharmacology | Pharmaceuticals |

<Learning Words>

A to Z	Dos and don'ts	Medication Online
Ask an Expert	Drug Online Database	Database
Ask a Pharmacist	Drug-related resources	Online information
Ask About Drugs	Drugs Online guides	

Detailed information on individual drugs or medications is often located at searchable online databases and directories maintained by pharmaceutical companies, industry associations, or medical schools. You find these by using the following magic search words:

<u>Drug Online Database</u>
<u>Medication Online Database</u>

Then search for the individual drug or medication you are interested in.

<Information Words>

| Biological unhappiness | Commonly used drugs | Contraindications |
| Brand-name medications | information | Dosage |

Drug interactions
Food and Drug
    Administration (FDA)
Generics
Indications
Lay person
Medication, medicines,
    drugs index

Natural health supplement
    guide
Overdose
Over the counter drugs
Patient Information
Pharmaceutical
Pharmacists Hotlines USA

Pharmacy
Precautions
Side effects
Warnings
Virtual Library Pharmacy
Vitamin and mineral
    supplement guide

<Medications>

Anti-arthritis drugs
Antispasmodic drugs
Bronchial therapy
Cardiovascular drugs
Cold medicines
Contraceptives
Cough medicines

Dermatological drugs
Diabetes therapy
Diuretics
Hormones
Nutrients
Ophthalmic preparations
Psychotherapeutic drugs

Sedatives
Strong analgesics
Supplements
Thyroid therapy
Treating Infections
Vitamins

<Medical Issue Words>

Acetominiphen
Allergic reactions
Allergy medicines
Anticholinergics
Antihistamines
Caffeine Interactions
Chemical composition
Chemicals
Choosing a pharmacy
Clinical trials
Cold and cough remedies
Communication with doctor
    and pharmacist
Contraindications

Cough suppressants
Dosing schedule
Driving
Drug abuse
Drug interactions
Drug overdose
Drug reactions
Drug safety
Drug therapies
Effects
Expectorants
Indications
Nasal decongestants

Overdose
Over the counter
Pain and fever medications
Prescriptions
Psychotherapeutic
Reading the labels
Safety with children
Saving money on drugs
Side effects
Sun Heat
Taking medication
Traveling with drugs
What to ask the doctor

<Types> Database

Analgesics
Antimicrobials
Antibiotics
Drug Classifications

Herbal medicine
Medications
Medicines

Muscle relaxants
Narcotics
Psychotropics

<Name> Information

Administration
Contraindications
Dosage

Indications
Interactions
Precautions

Proper use
Side effects
Warnings

<Phrase and Concept Words>

Avoiding the side effects of   Finding the right medicine   What medication should I
  <specific drug>   take

Examples:

medication side effects alternatives

antimicrobial use guidelines

your home medicine chest

herbal medicine chest

medicine cabinet safety

poisons in your home

synthroid side effects

precautions when taking drugs

driving while taking drugs

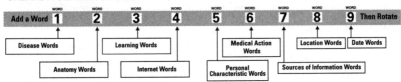

Men's Health

CREATE A SEARCH STRING

<Medical Specialties>

Internal medicine   Urology

<Learning Words>

A to Z   Because you are a man   Directories
Ask a doctor   Cool tools   FAQ's
Ask an Expert   Database   Q & A

<Information Words>

Diagnostic center   Fun with   Male reproductive system
  <location>   *<men's health issue>*   Man to man
Fun with *<disease>* Male diseases   Men for men
                    Male genital diseases

<Anatomy Words>

Bladder   Prostate   Testicles
Male reproductive organs   Scrotum   Urethra
Penis

<Medical Issue Words>

Circumcision   Disease information   Genital disease
Dating   Fitness   Hormones

Impotence

Men's health products

Prostate cancer

Infectious diseases

Overeating

Sexuality

Kidney

Patient Information

Substance abuse

Life expectancy

Pornography addiction

Testosterone

Masturbation

Premature ejaculation

Weight loss

Men's health problems

\<Disease Words\>

Bacterial infection

Penile growths

Sexual dysfunction

Cystitis

Penile injury

Stone disease

Epididymitis

Prostate disease

Testicular cancer

Fungal infection

Prostate cancer

Testicular torsion

Impotence

Priapism

Urethritis

Male infertility

Scrotal masses

Warts

Mumps

\<Medical Action Words\>

Alternatives

Identification

Quit smoking

Diagnosis

Immunization

Relationships

Early detection

Kicking bad habits

Self-examination

Family help

Prevention

Treatment *\<disease\>*

\<Phrase and Concept Words\>

Having a vasectomy

Questions to ask the doctor

Why am I impotent

Examples:

> understanding what's wrong with my sexual appetite
>
> men's health a to z
>
> testosterone diet
>
> dealing with prostate cancer
>
> fun with urology

Mental Health & Psychiatry

CREATE A SEARCH STRING

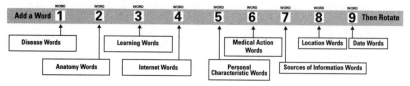

\<Medical Specialties\>

Psychology

Psychiatry

\<Learning Words\>

A to Z

Directories

Manuals

Ask an Expert

Patient information

Testing

Online Database

Guides

\<Information Words\>

Classification
Drug treatment
Mental disability

Mental disease
Mental examination

Mental health
Psychotherapy

\<Disease Words\>

Abnormal psychology
Abuse
Adolescence
Antidepressants
Alzheimer's disease
Antisocial
Anxiety attack
Anxiety disorders
Bed wetting
Bipolar disorders
Cult's deprogramming
Delusional disorder
Dementia
Dependant personality
  disorder
Depression
Dissociative disorders
Eating

Family problems
Fear
Gender identify
Hyperventilation
Learning disabilities
Mania
Marital problems
Mood Swings
Narcissistic
Neurosis
Obesity
Obsessive compulsive
  disorders
Phobic disorders
Pain
Panic attacks
Paranoia
Personality disorders

Psychosis
Phobias
Post trauma anxiety
Post traumatic stress
  disorders
Psychosexual disorders
Psychosomatic disorders
Psychotherapy
Relaxation
Schizophrenia
Seasonal Affective Disorder
Sexual disorders
Sleep disorders
Stress
Suicide
Tourette's Syndrome
Trauma

\<Medical Action Words\>

Alternatives
Assessment
Identification

Medication
Psychotherapy
Problem Identification

Therapy
Treatment

\<Medical Issue Words\>

Antidepressants
Anxiety
Combating stereotypes
Coping with stress
  inventory
Counseling
Counselors *\<location\>*
Dear Abby
Dear Anne Landers
Drugs
Drug treatment
Electro-shock treatment
Facts for *\<age\>*, *\<sex\>*,
  \<family relation\>
FAQ's Mental Health

Family history
Helping someone through
  *\<mental health
  disorder\>*
Inspirational
Medication
Meditation
Mental health fun
Mental health humor
Medical history
Mental measurements
Mind-body interaction
Online help mental health
Peace of mind
Personality tests

Physical examination
Psychotherapy
Self-help
Stress test
Surviving *\<specific mental
  health disorder\>*
Treatment *\<mental
  disorder\>*
Treatment centers
  \<location\>
Treatment saving money
Your questions answered
  *\<specific mental health
  disorder\>*

<Phrase and Concept Words>

Coping with mental disease   Dealing with depression   Finding the right doctor

Examples:

<u>surviving teenage mood swings</u>
<u>husbands surviving the first year of motherhood</u>
<u>husbands guide parenting humor</u>
<u>children post traumatic stress disorder violence</u>
<u>coping with divorce stress management</u>
<u>mental health treatment centers California Los Angeles</u>
<u>helping a person through a crisis</u>

Nervous System and Neurology

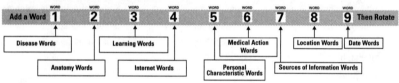

<Medical Specialties>

Neurology   Neurologists

<Learning Words>

A to Z   Ask a doctor   Ask an expert

<Information Words>

Caregivers	Nervous system	Physician locator
Evaluation	*<Anatomy Words>*	Resource centers
Information center	Nervous system *<biology>*	Tests
Mental status	Nervous system *<disease>*	Support centers
	Neurological examination	

<Anatomy Words>

Brain *<Anatomy Words>*	Brain Chemistry Layman	Spinal column
Brain *<disease>*	Nerves	

<Symptom Words>

Back pain	Hiccups	Stupor
Coma	Hypertension	Stuttering
Cramps	Nervousness	Tremor
Dizziness	Pain	Vertigo
Headache	Seizure	

Discovering the Fountain of Eternal Youth   101

<Disease Words>

Alzheimer's disease
Aneurisms
Attention deficit disorder
Autoimmune diseases
Carpal tunnel syndrome
Cerebral palsy
Chronic fatigue syndrome
Chronic illnesses
Coma
Delirium
Dementia

Encephalitis
Epilepsy
Headache
Head injuries
Huntington's disease
Movement disorders
Meningitis
Mental retardation
Multiple schlerosis
Muscular dystrophy

Parkinson's disease
Persian Gulf War syndrome
Repetitive strain injury (RSI)
Seizures
Smell disorders
Spine injuries
Stroke
Stupor
Taste disorders
Tumors

<Medical Issue Words>

Brain injury
Brain surgery
Diagnostic radiology
Encephalography
Head injury
Magnetic resonance
   imaging (MRI)

Neurological <disorders>
Neuro-toxicology
   information
Nuclear medicine
Positive emission
   tomography (PET)

Radiology
Spinal injuries
Spinal tap
Ultrasound
X-rays

<Medical Action Words>

Anesthetics
Assessment
Causes
Diagnosis
Diagnostic tests

Evaluation
Examination
Identification
Ergonomics
Medication

Prevention
Procedures
Referral service
Treatment
Therapy

<Phrase and Concept Words>

Dealing with
   <disease word>

Managing after a severe
   head injury

Preventing sports head
   injuries

Examples:

brain surgery information center
Alzheimer's disease family information resources
caring for people with Huntington's disease
treatment of pain alternatives

Physical & Developmental Disabilities

CREATE A SEARCH STRING

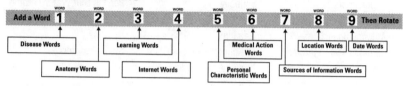

<Learning Words>

A to Z	Ask a doctor	Ask an expert

<Information Words>

ADA Information	Councils	Links
ADA Online	Disability <type> Resources	List servers
Adult care	Education	Mental retardation
Adult day care <location>	Government Information	Research
Associations	Information Center	Special Education
Caregivers		

<Medical Issue Words>

Americans with Disabilities Act	Facts for Families	Rehabilitation
Children who are mentally retarded	Legal issues	Sibling support
Communicative cognitive disabilities	Life planning for people with disabilities	Special camps
Disability Law	Parents helping parents	Special needs education
	Regional development centers	Special Olympics

Plastic Surgery

CREATE A SEARCH STRING

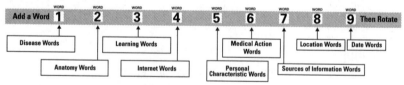

<Learning Words>

A to Z	Ask an expert	Possibilities
Ask a doctor	Guides	Questions and Answers
Ask a professional	Problems	Tutorials

<Information Words>

Centers <location>	Evaluating Qualifications	Institutes
Doctors	Plastic Surgeons	Making the decision

| Patient information | Patient support | Post operative advice |
| Patient rights | Patients | Preoperative advice |

\<Purposes>

Aesthetics	Hands	Obesity
Breast Implants	Head and Neck	Reconstructive
Burns	Liposuction	Teeth injuries
Cosmetic	Nose	Trauma
Facial		

\<Techniques>

| Grafting | Rhinoplasty |

\<Medical Action Words>

Alternatives	Recovery	Treatment
Examination	Rehabilitation	
Identification	Therapy	

Sex & Fertility

CREATE A SEARCH STRING

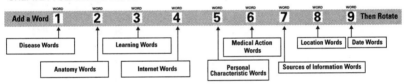

Be careful researching "sex" on the Internet. It is really easy to stumble into pornographic Web sites. You might wish to install a safe viewing program like NetNanny, or click on the safe viewing option available at many top search engines (e.g., Google.com)

\<Learning Words>

| A to Z | Ask a doctor | Resources |
| Ask an expert | Patient information | |

\<Information Words>

| Fertility | Pregnancy | Sexually transmitted |
| Infertility | | diseases |

\<Anatomy of Sexuality>

| Female reproductive | Male reproductive anatomy | Pregnancy |
| anatomy | Menstrual cycle | Reproduction genetics |

<Information Words>

A to Z
Ask an expert
Boys
Counseling
Databases
Directories

Girls
Guides
Interactive quizzes
Kids
Manuals

<age>
<gender>
<family relation>
<ethnic culture>
Teens

<Medical Issue Words>

Abortion
Abortion, types
AIDS & HIV Information
AIDS & HIV Prevention,
    Protection,
Birds and bees
Birth complications
Birth control
Birth control devices
Birth control pills

Care
Cervical caps
Communicating with
    parents
Condoms
Consensual
Contraception
Contraceptive foam or
    tablets
Contraceptive sponges

Counseling
Counseling centers
Counselors
Diagnosis
Diet
Drugs
Fertility
In vitro fertilization
Infertility *<sex>*

<Medical Action Words>

Alternatives
Infertility tests
Intrauterine devices (IUD's)
Lack of sexual desire
Natural family planning
Nonconsensual
Nutrition
Online tests
Peer Pressure
Positive sexuality
Post-coital contraception

Post-partem
Pregnancy
Pregnancy, high risk
Pregnancy, problems
Pregnancy, signs of
Pregnancy, special tests
Prenatal examinations
Reproductive rights
Rhythm method
Sex therapy

Sexual education legal
    issues
Spermacides
Sterilization men
Sterilization women
Teenagers safe sex
Travel
Treatment
Ultrasound
Withdrawal
X-rays

<Phrase and Concept Words>

Dealing with infertility
Finding help with

How do I know if

Where do I get help

Examples:

Seeking help with <Disease Word>
Dealing with Puberty
Dealing with Sticky situations
Preparing for childbirth
Preparing for pregnancy
Stages of childbirth
Stages of labor
Understanding masturbation

Sexual Disorders

CREATE A SEARCH STRING

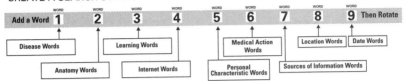

\<Medical Specialties\>

Internal Medicine
Psychiatry

Psychology

Urology

\<Learning Words\>

Ask About
Ask a doctor
Ask an Expert
Ask the Expert
Clearinghouse
Databases

Directories
Educational information
Epidemiological data
Fact sheets
FAQ's
Patient Information

Physician locator
Pocket guide to care
Q & A
Resource Centers
STD Clinic locator
Virtual Library

\<Symptom Words\>

Discharges
Genital growths
Nausea

Rashes
Ulcers

Vomiting
Weight loss

\<Anatomy Words\>

Female genitals
    \<Anatomy Words\>
Intestinal tract

Liver
Male genitals
    \<Anatomy Words\>

Skin

\<Disease Words\>

AIDS/HIV
Hepatitis
Herpes
Heterosexuality diseases

Homosexuality diseases
Mental health
Sexual dysfunction

Sexually transmitted
    diseases (STD's)
Viral Hepatitis

\<Medical Issue Words\>

Arousal
Behavior
Bisexual
Current events
Exhibitionism
Family members
Fetishes
Gay men disease risk
Gender identify disorders
Homosexuality

Inhibited orgasm
Late breaking news
Legal issues
Lesbian women disease risk
Low sexual desire
Masochism
Paraphiliac
Premature ejaculation
Related illnesses

Retarded ejaculation
Sadism
Sexual aversion disorder
Sexual dysfunctions men
Sexual dysfunctions women
Social issues
Support groups
Transsexual
Voyeurism

<Medical Action Words>

Alternative treatments	Medication	Therapy
Assessment	Prevention	Therapeutics
Causes	Quality of life	Transmission
Control	Role of the government	Treatment
Diagnosis	Surveillance	Vaccination
Identification	Testing	

<Phrase and Concept Words>

Dealing with sexual fetishes	Diagnosis of STD's	What you need to know about HIV

Examples:

medical management of HIV infection

can you get AIDS from kissing

planned parenthood AIDS/HIV information

prevention of STD's

AIDS/HIV incidence in Africa

what you need to know about AIDS

what children need to know about AIDS

living and coping with herpes

Skin Care and Skin Diseases

CREATE A SEARCH STRING

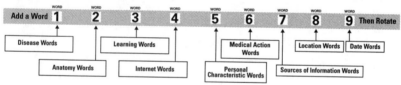

<Medical Specialties>

Common skin diseases	Dermatology	Skin care

<Learning Words>

A to Z	Ask an expert men	Ask an expert women
Ask a doctor		

<Anatomy Words>

Atrpophic skin	Epidermis	Nerve
Blister	Erosion	Nodules
Blood vessels	Fat layer	Sebaceous gland
Calluses	Growths	Scales
Corns	Hair follicle	Scar
Dermis	Hive	Skin

Subcutaneous tissue Sweat gland Wart

Sweat Ulcer Wheal

<Information Words>

Cosmetic companies Poisonous plants Solutions

Creams Powders Topical skin medications

Gels Skin care information Toxic substances

Lotions

<Disease Words>

Acne Impetigo Rosacea

Bacterial infections Infections Scabies

Bedsores Inflammation Scleroderma

Blisters Lice Sebaceous gland disorders

Calluses Lupus Shingles

Canker sores Male pattern baldness Skin cancer

Cellulitis Melanoma Sunburn

Corns Moles Sweatrng

Cysts Occupational skin diseases Tumors

Dermatitis Parasitic diseases Urticaria

Diabetics Pigment disorders Viral infections

Fever blisters Poison Ivy Viral warts

Fungal diseases Psoriasis Warts

Fungal infections Ringworm Worms

Hair loss

<Medical Action Words>

Diagnosis Management Plastic surgery

Identification Medications Treatment

<Symptom Words>

Bleeding Inflammation Scales

Blisters Itching Sore

Cold sores Pussy Spots

Discoloration Rashes Swollen

Hives Redness Whiteness

<Phrase and Concept Words>

Dealing with skin rash Treating bee stings What to do if you get badly burned

Examples:

<u>skin diseases caused by cosmetics</u>

<u>teenagers and acne treatment</u>

<u>genital warts prevention treatment</u>

<u>common bacterial infections of the skin diagnosis</u>

<u>skin diseases from sports</u>

<u>poison ivy treatment therapy</u>

Sleep Disorders

CREATE A SEARCH STRING

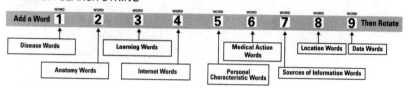

<Learning Words>
A to Z   Ask an Expert

<Information Words>
Accredited sleep   Sleep disorders   Sleep doctors
   laboratories *<location>*   *<Age Words>*   Sleep information
Daily sleep requirements Sleep disorders   Sleep laboratories
Sleep cycle normal   *<Gender Words>*   Sleep studies
Sleep disorders

<Disease Words>
Bed wetting   Narcolepsy   Sleep rocking
Bruxism   Nightmares   Sleep terrors
Fatigue   Night terrors   Sleepwalking
Fibromyalgia   Restless legs   Snoring
Head banging   Seasonal Affective Disorder Teeth grinding
Hypersomnia   Shift work   Wake cycle
Insomnia   Sleep apnea   Sleep cycle
Mood disorders   Sleep disorder syndromes

<Medical Issue Words>
Adolescence   Drugs   Psychological problems
Children   Image   School phobia
Death of parent   Infants   Self-esteem
Depression   Learning disabilities   Teens
Divorce   Mental health

<Medical Action Words>
Clinical test programs   Good habits   Self-help
Clinics   Medication   Self-tests
Diagnosis   Research centers   Treatment

<Phrase and Concept Words>
Getting help with sleep   How to help   How to stop
   disorders

Examples:

sleep disorders women treatment
how to stop snoring
accredited sleep labs Washington state

<u>do I have a sleep disorder?</u>
<u>sleep disorder research centers</u>
<u>sleepwalking diagnosis treatment</u>
<u>sleep management shift work preventing fatigue</u>
<u>proper use of Melatonin</u>

Social Problems, Physical, Sexual Problems

CREATE A SEARCH STRING

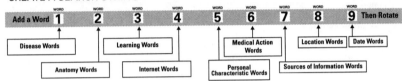

\<Medical Specialties\>

Mental health	Psychiatry	Psychology

\<Medical Issue Words\>

Addictions	Family problems	Rape
AIDS/HIV	Mental abuse	Sexual abuse
Alcohol abuse	Molestation	Substance abuse
Child abuse	Parental abuse	Teen pregnancy
Child pornography	Partner violence	Verbal abuse
Drug abuse	Physical Abuse	
Emotional abuse	Pornography addition	

\<Medical Action Words\>

Abuse Help lines	Emergency response	Hot lines
Care of	Family Help	Management
Caring for *\<family relation\>*	First Aid	Prevention
with *\<disease\>*	First responder	Therapy
Counseling	Guidance	Treatment
Emergencies	Help	

\<Phrase and Concept Words\>

How to deal with	What to do if	Where to get help

Examples:

<u>what to do if you've been raped</u>
<u>preventing spousal abuse</u>
<u>coping with mental abuse</u>
<u>dealing with parental abuse</u>
<u>prevention of child abuse</u>
<u>The role of parents</u>

Sports Medicine and Injuries

CREATE A SEARCH STRING

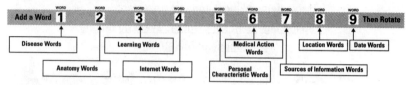

<Medical Specialties>
Orthopedics

<Information Words>

Ask a Doctor
Ask an Expert
Facility locator
Find a Doctor
Patient information

Physician locator
Running injuries
Sports injuries A to Z
Sports Injuries Index

Sports Medicine Database
Sports Medicine Directory
Sports Medicine online
Virtual hospital

<Medical Issue Words>

Coaches
Common sports injuries
Exercise injuries
Exercise programs

Injury prevention
Nutrition
Physical educators

Specialists
Trainers
Trauma disorders

<Symptom Words>

Broken bones
Fractures

Pain
Sprains

Strains
Swelling

<Common Athletic Injuries>

Achilles tendonitis
Hamstring injury
Runner's knee

Shin splints
Stress fractures
Tendonitis

Tennis elbow
Weight lifters back

<Anatomy Words>

Ligaments
Tendons

Knees
Hands

Elbows

<Medical Action Words>

Advice
Alternatives
Causes
Diagnosis

Management
Prevention
Rehabilitation
Relaxation

Stretching
Therapy
Treatment
Yoga

<Phrase and Concept Words>

Managing after a sports
    injury

Preventing sports injuries

What to do if

Examples:

<u>carpal tunnel syndrome surgery alternatives</u>

<u>bruises ice packs heating pads treatment</u>

<u>foot pain relief heel packs</u>

<u>androstenedione pros cons</u>

<u>aquatic therapy at home</u>

<u>home exercises for the stiff shoulder</u>

<u>yoga for the neck and shoulder</u>

Substance Abuse

CREATE A SEARCH STRING

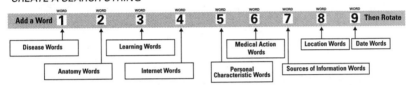

\<Information Words\>

A to Z	Ask an Expert	Manual
All about	Guide	Resources

\<Information Words\>

Addiction	Depressants	PCP
Alchohol	Designer drugs	Sleep aids
Amphetamines	Drug dependence	Speed
Anti-anxiety drugs	Hallucinogens	Stimulants
Biological effects	Inhalants	Street drug reference guide
Chemical abuse	Marijuana	Substance abuse
Cocaine abuse	Narcotic addictions	Uppers

\<Drug Abuse\>

Drug Abuse Assistance Education (D.A.R.E)	Drug policy information	Drug effects
Drug dependence	Drugs brain behavior	Resource Centers
Drug addiction	Drug tolerance	*\<location\>*
Drug Enforcement Administration (DEA) publications	Drugs prevention	
	Drug dependence	
	Drug education	
	Drug description	

\<Cultural Norms\>

Drugs *\<country\>*	Drugs *\<culture\>*

\<Crisis Intervention\>

Treatment centers *\<your location\>* City, County, State, Region	Treatment centers directory

<Special Resources>

Associations   National clearinghouse   National institute
Foundations   National council

<Alcohol>

Alcoholism   Drinking   Driving

<Smoking/Tobacco>

Alerts   Health and legal issues   Quit smoking
American Cancer Society   Hotlines   Second hand smoke
American Lung Association   Lung diseases prevention   Surgeon general reports
Anti-smoking advocates   Nicotine   Tobacco control
Cessation   Online consumer   Tobacco control advocates
Hazards of smoking   publications

<Marijuana Use>

Addiction   Fact sheets   Publications
Clearinghouse   Hazards   Real facts
Dangers   Prevention

<Phrase and Concept Words>

Anti-drug information   How to deal with   How to raise kids drug-free
Fight against   How to quit drugs   How to recognize
How to avoid

Surgery

CREATE A SEARCH STRING

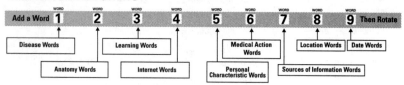

<Medical Specialties> <Surgeons>

Brain surgery   Internal medicine   Plastic surgery
Cardiac surgery

<Learning Words>

A to Z   Ask an expert   Problems
Ask a doctor   Guides   Questions and Answers
Ask a professional   Possibilities   Tutorials
Ask a surgeon

<Information Words>

Acceptance   Making the decision   Post-operative advice
Animations   Informed consent   Preoperative advice
Centers <*location*>   Institutes   Rejection
Doctors   Online atlas   Transplants
Evaluating Qualifications of   Patient support   Types of surgery
    Surgeons   Patients   Types of surgeons

<Purposes>

Aesthetics	Disease treatment	Injury
Brain	Emergency	Obesity
Cosmetic	Hands	Trauma
Facial	Head and Neck	Reconstructive
Burns	Internal	Rehabilitative
Cancer		

<Techniques>

Grafting	Laparoscopic	Surgery *<body part>*
Invasive procedures	Liposuction	Transplants
<body part>	Refractive	Vascular
Laser	Rhinoplasty	

<Medical Action Words>

Alternatives	Prognosis	Pre-operative care
Diagnosis	Medication	Treatment
Informed consent	Post-operative care	Therapy

<Phrase and Concept Words>

Finding a doctor	What to ask the doctor	What you need to know

Examples:

Before you have surgery

Surgery and informed consent

Questions to ask your doctor

How long have you been performing surgery

Talking to your doctor

What you should know before surgery

Preparing for surgery

Preoperative information for patients

Help for healing

Tests, Tools and Calculators

CREATE A SEARCH STRING

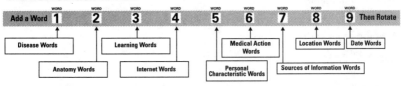

There are an ever-increasing number of online tests, tools and calculators that allow people to analyze and examine a wide variety of health conditions. They range from simple to sophisticated.

You can use magic search words to learn all about specific diagnostic tests your doctor may be prescribing for you or find online tests that act as an extension of an actual examination, measurement or evaluation.

Many of the online tests are self-help tests designed for lay people to identify their risk or need for action with respect to an illness or condition.

<Diagnostic Tests>

Blood tests	Muscular system	Skeletal system
Cancer tests	Neurological system	Specimen tests
Circulatory System	Reproductive system	Thyroid system
Digestive System	Respiratory system	Urinary system

<Internet Words>

Interactive	Online	Survey

<Learning Words>

Patient information	Self-help	Tests
Risk	Self-test	Understanding

<Specific Health or Medical Tests>

Anger anxiety	Eating disorder	Resilience
Biopsy tests	Evaluating chest pain	Self-esteem
Burnout	Heart attack survival	Sensory motor
Cancer	Heart problems	Sleep
Coping skills	Lifestyle	Speech
Depression	Nutrition	Vision

<Mental Health>

Achievement tests	Medical trivia Tests	Tests, personality tests,
Behavior assessment	Mental tests	psychological testing
Developmental	Neuro-physiological	
IQ Tests	Personality tests	
Medical trivia test challenges	Self assessments, quizzes, tests	

<Tools> <Calculators>

Clinical calculators	Medical calculators	Metric converters

<Specific Tools or Calculators>

Basal metabolism	Daily food planners	Fat or fiction
Blood alcohol	Depression	Food
Body mass index	Diet calculators	Health risk assessment
Calories, caloric requirements, fat, protein, carbohydrates, sodium, protein, fiber,	Dietary recommendations Disease Environmental	Healthy Body, eat well Ideal weight Nutrient database

Nutritional value, *<Food>*,   Risk assessment   Safe Food
    <Fast food> example,   Risk reports   Vitamin ABC's
    nutritional value content
    hamburger McDonald's

Examples:

<u>Men test your knowledge of women</u>
<u><Sex> test your knowledge of <opposite sex></u>
<u>Test your knowledge of sexual problems</u>
<u>Test your knowledge of <subject></u>

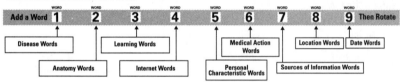

Travel and Health

CREATE A SEARCH STRING

| Add a Word | WORD 1 | WORD 2 | WORD 3 | WORD 4 | WORD 5 | WORD 6 | WORD 7 | WORD 8 | WORD 9 | Then Rotate |

Disease Words — Learning Words — Medical Action Words — Location Words — Date Words

Anatomy Words — Internet Words — Personal Characteristic Words — Sources of Information Words

<Information Words>
Travel medicine patient information   Travel planning medical health information

<Travel Health Issues>

Allergies	Heart attacks	Strokes
Allergies	Hyperventilation	Sunlight
Asthma	International travel	Temperature
Blowing dust	Medications	Ultraviolet light
Diabetes	Migraine	Vaccinations
Headaches	Pollution	Vision
Health meteorology	Seasonal affective disorder	Weather effects
Health weather	Skin	*<body parts>*

<Medical Action Word>
Coping with   Managing   Treatment
Dealing with

<Phrase and Concept Words>
Finding safe drinking water   What to do if   Where to get help in

Examples:

<u>How the weather affects your health</u>
<u>Preventing hypothermia</u>
<u>Dealing with Heat stroke</u>
<u>Allergies and air quality</u>
<u>Aches and Pains and changing weather</u>
<u>Protecting your skin from the sun</u>

Women's Health

CREATE A SEARCH STRING

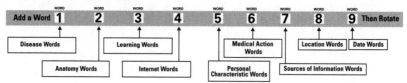

<Medical Specialties>

Gynecology	Obstetrics	Urology

<Learning Words>

Ask questions	Ask a Doctor Woman	FAQ's
	<disease>	Questions and answers

<Information Words>

External genital organs	Fun with Women *<disease>*	Menstruation
Facts about Women	Gynecological examination	Puberty
<disease>	Hormones	Reproduction
Female genital organs	Internal genital organs	Straight Talk about Women
Female reproductive system	Menopause	*<disease>*

<Anatomy Words>

Breasts	Pelvis	Vulva
Female reproductive system	Vagina	

<Medical Issue Words>

Abortion	Choosing an obstetrician/	Mammograms
Aging	gynecologist	Mastectomy
Baby feeding	Contraception	Mental health
Baby growth and	Delivery options	Midwife
development	Domestic violence	Pregnancy
Because you are a woman	Exploring women's health	Puberty
<health issue>	Family planning	Surgery alternatives
Breast feeding with	Feminist Health women	Teen pregnancy
implants	Information for women	The gynecological
Breast Feeding, lactation	*<medical specialty>*	examination
Caesarian section	Information for women	Woman to woman, Women
Cancer	OB/GYN	to women
Child birth		

<Disease Words>

Abnormal bleeding	Breast cancer clear	Breast cancer tutorial
AIDS/HIV	explanations	layperson
Arthritis	Breast cancer early	Breast disorders
Breast cancer treatment	detection	Breast lumps
options		

Breast pain
Cancer *<type>*
    <action word>
Candiasis
Chlamydial infections
Crabs
Cracked hands skin care
Cysts
Delivery
Disease complications
Eating disorders
Ectopic pregnancy
Eczema
Endometriosis
Fallopian tubes
Fertility, infertility
Fetal alcohol syndrome
Fibrocystic disease
Fibroids
Genetic disorders
High risk pregnancy

Infections
Infertility
Inhibited orgasm
Irritable bladder
Lice
Low sex desire disorders
Mastitis
Menopause
Menstruation
Menstrual disorders
Miscarriages
Nipple discharge
Osteoporosis
Ovarian cancer
Ovarian disorders
Ovulation
Ovulation method
Parasites
Pelvic inflammatory disease
Pelvic pain

Polycistic ovaries
Premature menopause
Premenstrual syndrome
Prolapse
Sexual arousal disorders
Sexual disorders
Skin problems
    <action word>
Stress incontinence
Toxic shock syndrome
Tumors
Urologic disorders
Vaginal disorders
Vaginal infections
Vaginal odor
Vaginitis
Vulvitis
Varicose veins
Warts
Yeast infections

<Medical Action Words>

Causes
Diagnosis
Evaluation
Examination
Homeopathic Care

Homeopathic Products
Identification
Medication
Prevention therapy
Screening

Surgery
Tests
Therapy
Treatment
Treatment Alternatives

<Symptom Words>

Abdominal swelling
Abnormal bleeding
Absence of menses
Amenorrhea
External genitalia pain
Irritation

Itching
Lower abdominal pain
Lower back pain
Menstrual cramps
Mittelschmerz
Painful intercourse

Pelvic pressure
Premenstrual tenderness
Urinary incontinence
Vaginal discharge
Vaginal protrusion

<Phrase and Concept Words>

Dealing with

Finding a doctor

Getting help

Examples:

Dealing with <condition>
Do's and don'ts
Managing during <illness>
Preparing for <disease>

<u>Shopping medicine saving money</u>
<u>Specific Products by name (e.g., Tampons)</u>
<u>because you are a woman pregnancy discrimination</u>
<u>breast cancer treatment alternatives</u>
<u>managing menopause</u>
<u>homeopathy skin problems</u>
<u>dealing with pms</u>
<u>sexual arousal disorder therapy alternatives</u>

X-rays, Radiology and Nuclear Medicine

CREATE A SEARCH STRING

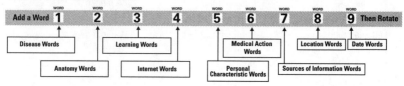

<Medical Specialties>

Diagnostic radiology	Radiology	Radiologist

<Learning Words>

A to Z	Ask a doctor	Dictionaries
Ask about	Database	Resources
Ask an expert	Directories	

<Information Words>

MRI Image Maps	Ultrasound obstetrics	Virtual medical library
nuclear medicine layman	Virtual medical center	x-rays understanding

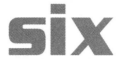

The Castles of the Kingdom

Go after the organizations and institutions that have the information or offer the services you need or want the most.

Go after organizations that are located where you live or are in places where you want to be.

Study the categories and magic search words below and identify the specific categories or topics that you are interested in.

There are special techniques you can use to pursue and acquire information from the special sources that are described in this section.

You will use the *<Information Source Words>* for your particular search. These become magic search words for your search strings.

Rotate through the *<Source Words>* you identify, searching for information that will help you reach your goal.

Going from Ideas to Action

Remember you are on a search with a special purpose. Once you identify a medical treatment opportunity or direction you may need to take action and implement it.

To do this, you must have the essential information about what exactly you need—who offers it, what it is, where it is, and how do you get it. This is the reality end of the business of health care business.

This is the critical business information you are after.

Once you have this information you can seek to acquire the information, products or services you need.

The Importance of Finding Critical Business Information (CBI)

You have to take everything you've learned and focus it on really going for the gold. By searching for specific health care service providers we are about to put ideas into action.

Think of yourself as on a treasure hunt, searching for golden nuggets of information. You will capture these golden nuggets and turn them into real gold.

The Internet offers you access to expert information, news about companies, governments, organizations, and contact information. The primary goal of your whole Internet search effort focuses on uncovering "Critical Business Information" or CBI for short.

This is what you are ultimately after. Your search boils down to looking for:

(i)   Who to contact;
(ii)   What is the actual specific information or opportunity;
(iii)   Where the opportunity is located; and
(iv)   How you have to apply or qualify for the opportunity.

Properly utilized, the critical intelligence forms the basis for action that can result in you finding and applying for health care or service. You have to know *how* to look, and you have to know *what* to look for—and you also have to *know* it when you *see* it.

It really isn't hard. Most people who are hungry for information have "situational awareness" and they instinctively know critical business information when they see it or hear it:

CBI is easy to spot when you see it or hear it. Just look for the who, what, where, when, and how.

However, CBI is not that always easy to come by. It is disguised and buried in layers of Web pages and bureaucracy. Sometimes you have to investigate a little further or be inventive to create a missing piece of critical information.

What you really need to turn CBI into real opportunity is "how" to get what you want.

The Classical Use of Conventional CBI

Before the Internet, people searching for health care information had to use paper sources of information.

They read newspapers, went to libraries, and visited government reading rooms for trade publications and other specialized materials all in pursuit of identifying those little tidbits of critical business information.

To get contact information people had to use telephone books, and huge, often out-dated, printed directories, by talking with employees, secretaries, human relations personnel, and librarians.

And it worked for them.

When people heard about an opportunity, they took action. They called by phone, wrote a letter and sent for written information or sent in an application. They called or went to see the person offering the health care service or provider opportunity.

Traditionally it took a long, long time.

The New Way to Get CBI

The processes and the tools and the skills people used before the Internet are still the same as you use now.

Sure, there are a few innovations-like Internet communications and e-mail, but these are basically just technological conveniences.

Realize this—they are simply advances in the technology of communication. Society has seen advances before: the mail to phone, phone to fax, fax to Internet, and most recently from Internet to wireless.

People continue to research to get information, but now the time it takes is shorter. They read written words in a greater variety of forms. They can exercise communications across a much wider network with other people, conducting informational interviews to find CBI.

Today, with the vast resources of the Internet and e-mail, this can be accomplished faster, easier and cheaper than ever before.

However, to apply and negotiate these opportunities, you still need to make phone calls, write letters, and send in applications, letters, and conduct interviews. You still have to complete written applications and transmit them.

All this is still true. The actual search and decision-making processes that people go through is still the same.

It is up to you to take these actions.

Special Topics in Medical Health Care

Medicine is in the most dramatic period of technological advance the world has ever seen. The methods used to identify, diagnose and treat disease are changing rapidly and extensively. Not only are there new diagnostic tests, medications, and therapies, but the face of health and medical care and the nature of the institutions that provide care is also in a state of constant renovation.

The Internet represent an incredible opportunity for both medical health practitioners and patients. The Internet provides an efficient vehicle for improved professional and patient education and information.

The patient-physician relationship can be improved with better communication, education and knowledge.

Use the Internet and Magic Search Words to fill in your need for knowledge and understanding of the medical health care system. Learn how to use it and avoid being abused by it.

Understanding more about the health care system and the types of care different facilities offer can minimize your stress in dealing with the system and save you time and money in getting the right care you need.

Use Magic Search Words and learn how to make better use of the health care resources that are available to you.

Topic	Page
Doctors & Health Care Professionals	123
Hospitals and Health Care Facilities	124
Insurance & Health Care	125
Medical Education	126
Government Agencies	127
Companies and Corporations	128
Professional Associations & Organizations	129
Educational Institutions	131
Media	132
Legal Questions and Fraud or Abuse	134
Free Stuff	135

Doctors & Health Care Professionals

Learn about doctors and other health care professionals you encounter

<Levels of Care>

Primary Care	Secondary care	Tertiary Care

<Medical Doctors>

A to Z	Directory	Training
Continuing education	Medical schools	Types of doctors

<Nurses>

A to Z	Directory	Training
Continuing Education	Nursing schools	Types of nurses

<Health-Care Professionals>

Dental hygienists	Nurses aids and attendants	Physician assistants
Emergency medical technicians (EMT's)	Occupational therapists	Podiatrists
	Opticians	Psychologists
Home health aids	Optometrists	Radiologic technicians
Licensed practical nurses (LPN's)	Orthotists and Prosthetists	Radiologists
	Paramedics	Recreational therapists
Medical records personnel	Pharmacists	Registered dietitians
Medical technologists	Physical Therapists	Respiratory therapists

Social Workers   Speech pathologists and
                          audiologists

<Information Words>

Ask a Doctor   Medical definitions   Questions to ask doctor
Ask the Doctor *<specialty>*   Questions for doctor   before surgery
Ask the Expert   *<specialty>*   Specialties
Disciplines   Specialties database

<Issues>

Changing doctors   Concerns about doctors   Evaluating doctors
Choosing a doctor   Consulting doctors online Getting a second opinion
Choosing a surgeon   Frequently asked questions Selecting a doctor
Comparing doctors   Consumer questions

<Aids>

Find a doctor   Physician Locators   Referral services
Find a surgeon   Quackwatch   Selecting a doctor

<Phrase and Concept Words>

Ask your doctor   Getting the most out of   What questions to ask

Example:

<u>Checking a doctor's qualifications</u>
<u>Getting the most out of your doctor</u>
<u>Communicating with your doctor</u>
<u>How to get a second opinion</u>
<u>Talking with your doctor</u>
<u>Verify credentials of a doctor</u>
<u>Avoiding medical fraud</u>
<u>find a psychologist</u>
<u>find a dentist</u>
<u>find a anesthesiologist</u>

Hospitals and Health Care Facilities

Learn about hospitals and health care

<Kinds of Hospitals>

Ambulatory surgical centers   General hospitals   Profit hospitals
Community health centers   Medical centers   Public hospitals
Community hospitals   Non profit hospitals   Teaching hospitals
Freestanding emergency   Private hospitals
centers

\<Parts of the Hospital\>

Cardiology
Coronary care
Critical care
Emergency room
Intensive care
Maternity

Neonatal intensive care
Neurology
Nuclear medicine
Oncology
Outpatient department
Physical therapy

Pulmonary
Radiology
Rehabilitation
Shock trauma
Social services

\<Issues\>

Accreditation
Admission procedures
Elective surgery
Home care

Hospices
Outpatient surgery
Preoperative routines
Prepping

Recovery
Special facilities
The operation

\<Quality of Hospital Care\>

Arbitration
Malpractice
Patient's rights

Patient's role in the hospital
Remedying deficient
   hospital care

What to do in case of death

\<Special Information\>

Consumers guide
Health care handbook

Manual guide
Patient bill of rights

Patient guide
Patient rights

\<Phrase and Concept Words\>

Checklists doctors office
How to handle staying in
   hospital

Is hospitalization
   necessary?
Overnight in the hospital

Visits to the hospital
What to expect during your
   stay

Insurance & Health Care

Learn about who pays for medical health care and insurance.

\<Insurance & Payment\>

Employee health plans
Health care
Health maintenance
   organization (HMO)

Health plans
Medicaid
Medical and hospital
   insurance

Medicare
Preferred provider
   organizations (PPO)
Prepaid health plans

\<Issues\>

Comparing insurance
Evaluating insurance

Evaluating the adequacy of
   your coverage
How to

Selecting insurance
   coverage
Tutorials

\<Information\>

Appeals, grievances
Consumer advocacy
Diagnostic related groups
Facility locators

Health/Medical/Dental
   insurance, shopping for,
   comparing, evaluating

Hospice care, Medicare,
   Medicaid
Managed Care

Medical records
Patient advocacy
Plan limits, catastrophic
   coverage, home health,
   exclusions, dental, eye
   care, long term care
   features, free care,
   charity care,

<Government>

Complaints, abuse, fraud,
   watchdog, whistleblower

Policy, legislation,
   congressional
   testimony, court
   decisions, litigation,
   lawsuits
Programs, quality, features,
   costs, benefits

Government, US, State

Public care, private care
Reasonable costs
Select, choose, compare,
   geographic location,
   network
Seniors & children

Medical Education

<General Medical Resources>

Advice
Anatomy & Physiology
   database
Anatomy education
Biological education
Biomedical education
Case studies
Counseling, counselors
Cures, treatments, teaching,
   teaching cases
Fun Stuff
General medical education
Health education

Imaginary patient play
   doctor
Information Education
   Layperson
Information pages
Interactive patient
Learning all about
   <disease>
Links
Medical Discoveries
Medical humor
Medical interactive
   discovery

Medical interactive learning
Medical Mysteries, medical
   mysteries solved, humor
Medical myths
Patient education
Resources
Science, science fiction,
Self-help
Teaching patients all about
   <disease>
Tips

<Health Information Resources>

A to Z index
Acronyms
Animations
Cellular biology
Cross-sections

Dictionaries
Encyclopedias
Illustrations
Interactive self-assessment
Matrix

Microbiology
Nobel Prize medicine,
   physiology
Pharmacology
Pictures

<Anatomy resources>

Anatomy *<body part>*
Brain chemistry layman
Cyberpatient
Digital anatomist *<body
   part>*
Dissections *<body part>*
Embryo development
   pictures
Forensic science

Histological photographs
Human anatomy online
Human body virtual project
Human simulation
Human viewer
Illustrations
Image archives
Images of bacteria
Images of viruses

Interactive patient care
   simulator
Medical images of the brain
Multimedia tutorials
Online exploration
   <body part>
Online interactive atlases
Pathology slides
Physiology online

Pictures of bacteria
Sources of images and
animations
Step-by-step dissections

Tutorials <*body part*>
Virtual anatomy
Virtual medical center
Virtual medical library

Visible female
Visible human cross
sections
Visible male

<Environmental Health>

Chemicals effects on
humans
Children's health
environmental
Environmental medicine

Household hazards
How safe is your home
Indoor air pollution
Outdoor air pollution
Radiation effects on

humans
Solutions for a health home
Stratospheric ozone

<Genetics & Biotechnology>

Biotechnology information
Chromosome locations
Education centers
Ethical, legal, social issues

Gene maps
Genetic counselors
Genetic disease treatment

Genetic disorders
Human genome project
information

Government Agencies

Government agencies have huge resources that continue getting better and better. You access them by entering the magic search word "government" plus the <*Learning Words*> and <*Internet Words*>.

Examples:

<u>US government online directories</u>
<u>US government online databases</u>
<u>US government agencies searchable index</u>

Government <Source>

A to Z
Agencies by state
Agencies by name
Directories

Databases
Locators
Personnel locators
Servers

Specialized databases
Specialized directories
Telephone directories

Government <Type>

International
National
Country

Federal
State
Regional

County
City
Local

Government <Branch>

Executive agencies
Legislative branch
Congress

House of Representatives
Congressional offices

Judicial offices
Governors

Government <Geography>

Country	Province	County
State	Region	City

Government <Subject>

You can also find government agencies by searching on the subject for which they are responsible:

Agriculture	Employment	Natural resources
Air	Energy	Regulations
Airlines	Environment	Safety
Aviation	Health	Small business
Business	Housing	Soil conservation
Communications	Income	Statistics
Courts	Labor	Taxes
Crime	Laws	Telecommunication
Cultural	Legal	Transportation
Demographics	Libraries	Water
Economic	Medicine	Welfare
Education		

Companies and Corporations

Medical equipment	Laboratory services	Pharmaceutical

<Companies> <Corporations>

You can search for companies by using *<Learning Words>* and *<Internet Words>* along with the following words:

<Types>

Businesses	Corporations	Services
Companies	Manufacturers	Consulting

Examples:

<u>online directory business</u>
<u>online database medical companies</u>
<u>software companies a to z</u>

Industry <Source>

A to Z	Directories	Specialized databases
Associations by name	Locators	Specialized directories
Association by state	Personnel locators	Telephone directories
Databases	Servers	

<Industry>

Industry group	Industry classification	Standard industrial code
Industry by name	system	SIC code

You can also search for companies by industry and by geography or location.

Company <Industry> <Location>

Known or general location	Region	County
Country	State	City

<Actual Company Name>

You can also search for an association by its actual name. When you find the individual company Web sites, you can look for people who can give you information about what you are looking for.

Executives	Departments	Membership
Offices	Divisions	Chapters

Company <News>
Company <Media Centers>

You can find out a lot of information about companies by visiting online media press centers. There you can view and often search for:

News releases	Industry news	Competition information
Press releases	Competitor information	

News releases almost always contain contact names and phone numbers of senior executives, or public relations or external affairs personnel. Contact these people directly and ask them specific questions about whom you should contact to find out more about health and medical information.

Professional Associations & Organizations

Professional health organizations, associations, and private non-profit institutions have huge online resources that continue getting better and better. You access them by entering the *<Association or Organization Words>* plus the *<Learning Words>* and *<Internet Words>*.

Examples:

<u>associations online directories</u>
<u>organizations online databases</u>

Select magic search words from other word groups and combine them with *<Association Words>* like this:

<Disease> <Association Word>
<type of doctor> <Association Word>
<medical specialty> <Association Word>
<location> <Association Word>
<nationality> <Association Word>

Here are a list of *<Association or Organization Words>*

<Association Words>

Academy	Government, human	Professional organizations
Alliances	services, health services	Research centers
Associations	Information centers	Resource centers
Brotherhoods	Institutes	Sisterhoods
Centers	National Institutes	Societies
Clinics	Networks	Sororities
College	Nonprofit organizations	Support groups
Community connections	Online communities of/for	Trade organizations
Councils	patients	University
Federations	Organizations	Workgroups
Foundations	Organizations	Workshops
Fraternities	Professional associations	

Examples:

American Cancer Society
National Clearinghouse Drug Prevention
National Institutes Health Searchable Database Medicine
Mental health support groups
Sleep disorder research centers
American Diabetes Association

Associations and professional trade organizations often are identified by fraternal words, go by many names and can be searched in a number of ways.

Associations <Types>

Academic	Industry	Social
Advocacy	Labor	Technical
Art	Political	Trade
Cultural	Research	

Once you are on an association Web site, you look for key information sources using the following words:

<Information Sources>

A to Z	Databases	Servers
Association by state	Directories	Specialized databases
Chapters by location	Locators	Specialized directories
Chapters by name	Personnel locators	Telephone directories

You can also search associations by industrial codes.

Associations <Industry>

Industry by name	system	SIC code
Industry classification	Industry group	Standard industrial code

You can also search for industry by geography or location.

Association <Industry> <Geography>

Known or general location	Region	County
Country	State	City

<Actual Association by Name>

You can also search for association by their actual name. Once at an association web site you can find specific resources and information including:

Executives	Membership	Chapters
Offices		

You can also search associations by the type of events they put on.

<Events>

Events represent special opportunities to identify and meet with people. Search for them and go to them.

Conferences	Seminars	Training
Conventions	Symposiums	Workshops
Meetings	Trade shows	

Educational Institutions

<Colleges>	**<Universities>**	**<High Schools>**

Colleges and universities have huge health resources that get better and better. You access them by entering the *<Education Word>* plus the *<Learning Words>* and *<Internet Words>*.

Examples:

<u>schools online directories</u>
<u>universities online databases</u>
<u>colleges searchable index</u>

Once you get to specific university Web sites, you identify and look for health information.

College or University <Source>

A to Z	Directories	Specialized databases
School listings by name	Locators	Specialized directories
School listings by state	Personnel locators	Telephone directories
Databases	Servers	

Once you are on an educational institution Web site you can find a whole world of specific resources and information.

You must study and learn how to navigate the Web sites you find, as each one will be unique and different.

Media

Media Web sites often have specialized directories, databases or search engines which allow you access to vast archived articles on key subjects of interest to you.

You can read and learn about your areas of interest.

You access them by entering the *<Media Word>* plus the *<Learning Words>* and *<Internet Words>*.

A to Z	Locators	Servers
By format	Media by location	Specialized databases
Call letter	Media by name	Specialized directories
Databases	Media by state	Telephone directories
Directories	Personnel locators	

The key search strings to use are:

<u>\<Medical Topic\> \<Media Category\></u>
<u>\<Medical Topic\> \<Media Category\> \<Media People\> \<Illness\></u>
<u>\<Disease\> \<Type Of Media Publication\></u>
<u>\<Disease\> \<Specific Issue\> \<Type Of Media Publication\></u>

Examples:

<u>media online database</u>
<u>media online directory</u>

Once you use media directories and databases you can go to an individual media Web site and then search for specific information.

Media <Types>

Cable shows	Newspapers	Trade publications
Cable systems	Radio networks	TV networks
Daily newspapers	Radio shows	TV shows
Magazines	Radio stations	TV stations
News networks	Radio syndicates	TV syndicates
News services	Tabloid newspapers	Weekly newspapers
News syndicates		

Media <Industry Categories>

You can search on media industry categories in a number of ways. There are very extensive searchable and specialized directories and databases online.

You can identify the names, classifications or categories of industry that you are interested in and then search for the media that cover that topic.

Find them by searching using the *<Learning words>* and the *<Internet Words>* with various specific industry names, categories or classifications, along with the media terms above. Some of the key media categories covering health include:

Chemical	General interest	Medical
Computers	Government	Men's magazines
Conservation and ecology	Health and fitness	Parenting
Cosmetics	Healthcare	Pets and animals
Dentistry	Home and garden	Pharmacy
Education	Hotel, motel and hospitality	Science
Environmental	Insurance	Women's
Funeral		

Media <Specialty Editors>

Media specialty editors are responsible for generating the news or articles you read on a certain topic. You can search for them by name or title. They often go by one of the following titles, along with their particular area of specialty.

| Editors | Columnists | Specialty |
| Reporters | Correspondents | |

You can select the specialty from this list:

Beauty / Grooming	Family / Parenting	Medical
Book Review	Fitness and exercise	Medical Business
Computers / High Tech	Food	Medical / Health
Consumer Interest	Health	Nutrition
Education / Higher	Home	Science
Education	Internet	Seniors / Retirement
Environmental	Investments	Women
Exercise / Fitness	Lifestyle	

Examples:

<u>Medical health magazines</u>
<u>Medical health columns</u>
<u>Medical health columnist</u>
<u>Men's health columnist</u>
<u>Athletic injury prevention articles</u>
<u>Doctors featured articles osteoporosis</u>
<u>Diabetes featured articles</u>
<u>Diabetes self-management featured articles</u>
<u>Children illness self-management online articles</u>

Legal Questions and Fraud or Abuse

Consumer advocacy groups, institutions and individuals stand ready to help you guard against waste, fraud and abuse.

You can search to find information to help you avoid health abuse by searching on the following:

Alchemists	Health-related frauds, fads,	Medical Scams
Avoiding quacks and	myths and fallacies	Pseudoscience
misinformation	Heretics	Quackwatch
Busting quacks and frauds	How to recognize quacks	Quality of health
False advertising, mail	and frauds	information on the
order, products	Medical Abuse	Internet
Fines and penalties	Medical and surgical	Questionable medical
Fraud Task Force	malpractice consultants	devices
Health professionals	Medical Fraud	Watchdogs, watchtowers
litigation alerts	Medical malpractice suits	Whistleblowers
Health superstitions	Medical Quacks,	

Free Stuff

The Internet has developed a culture where quality information is free, most of the time. If you don't want to pay, keep on looking for the free resources. To zero in on free resources, use the following magic search words in your search strings:

Booklet	Help	Strategies
Bulletin board	Help centers	Tactics
Do's and don'ts	Manual	Test
E-mail consultations	Online manual	Tips
Forum	Quiz	Tutorial
Guide	Self help	

CREATE A SEARCH STRING

WORD	WORD	WORD	WORD	
Add a Word **1**	**2**	**3**	**4**	**Then Rotate**

Subject Words
Disease Words
Medical Issue Words
Symptom Words
Medical Actions Words

Learning Words
All About
A to Z
Database
Directory
Information
Tutorial

Internet Words
Online
Searchable
Center
Virtual
Supersite

Source Words
Government
Business
Community
Organizations
Educational Institutions
Associations

seven

Conclusion

Hopefully, with the help of this *Magic Search Words* book, you will have learned to search for information on the Internet that will improve your life.

As you go out and search for information, read with the purpose of using it right away.

Read for critical information. Plan on using it.

Be proactive with the information that you find.

Take action. Make sure that you use what you find.

Don't stop till you achieve success.

Avoiding Disaster

Identify and avoid medical scams, fraud and abuse. If it seems to good to be true, it definitely is.

There are well known warning signs you can use to identify a likely scam:

- If they say it'll cost you money to match and find you a insurance or medical services, it's probably a scam.
- If they say, they just need your credit card to hold the services for you, it's probably a scam.
- If they say it's guaranteed and they'll do all the work for you, it's probably a scam.
- If they seek to charge you for just a service fee, it's probably a scam.

Don't get taken for a bum ride. Learn how to identify scams and fraudulent schemes. Do a search on the words:

MEDICAL SCAMS FRAUD

Study up on how to avoid getting caught in a scam. Learn what the government and watchdog agencies say about how to recognize a medical scam and qualify a search service.

Protect yourself.

How Good Is the Magic?
GIGO (Garbage in Garbage Out) or MIMO (Magic In, Magic Out)

You must evaluate the quality of the information on the web sites you find constantly. Before you assume that information is valid and factually correct, you should:

1. Determine its source origin. Discover the author, the publisher and the purpose of the web site.
2. Are they objective, unbiased, and independent? Or are they selling products or services? Do they have ulterior motives?
3. Determine the authors and publisher's credentials, expertise, and experience. Do the author's qualifications support their ability to provide factually correct information?
4. Identify the date of the writing to establish the historical context.
5. Verify it. Find at least one other reputable source that provides similar substantiating information.

Learn more about how to assess the quality and truthfulness of information on the Internet. Search on:

evaluating the quality of information on the Internet checklist
assessing the quality of web sites information
identifying fraudulent, inaccurate and questionable web sites
quality of information on the Internet
criteria for evaluating web site information

Parting Words

People often ask. "What is the best way to search on the Internet?"

Use search strings.

But please remember that the real answer to the question depends on what you are willing and able to do.

What you search, find and apply for will depend on your wants and interests, and the time and energy you invest in the effort. Only you can determine what you want, need and are willing to do to get it.

Even if you search just a few times and find some interesting and useful information, you can keep on searching and find more and different and potentially even more useful information.

If you stop searching, one thing is for certain, you'll get nothing more. If you continue searching, finding and learning, the odds are in your favor that you'll understand a whole lot more.

Fortunately, the Internet and search engines have evolved so that information to help you find what you are looking for is right at your fingertips.

Search. Learn the key search techniques and become proficient at them.

Start searching. Do it and do it now. You have nothing to lose and a world of health information to gain.

Once you start, this is what will happen:

- You will discover and release a desire to find and utilize new resources within yourself. You will suddenly want to achieve new things in your life.
- You will become more knowledgeable, more competent, better trained, more creative, more skilled, and more adventurous.

- You will learn new things. You will come up with new ideas that will help you replace old self-defeating patterns of behavior and boredom. You will be able to use the new information, and improve yourself with new tool, skills and abilities.
- You will realize that knowledge is power. At every step, you will learn something new and something powerful.

What you can expect:
- You will act on that information and come closer to your goal.
- You will understand that the key to success in life is to take action on what you learn.

As you act, you trigger actions in others, and new information and new opportunities will come your way. Don't hesitate—act on them.

As you experience the thrill of creating these opportunities, you will develop a sense of wonder and respect for knowledge and a love and appreciation for learning.

Believe in creative reality. Make your dreams come true. Do it.

Search. Start your search knowing what you want. Visualize it as best you can.

Look at the steps in this book as a way to reach within yourself and use the amazing Internet resources that are available at your fingertips to create a new vision and a new reality for your life.

This book can help you make your searching time and efforts more efficient and effective so that it is really worth your time and effort.

Don't get hooked on relying on the monster medical search databases alone. There is a lot of material written that does not get into the specialized databases.

You learn more by searching yourself and taking the actions needed to get more information directly from the source. You will be surprised that most of this information will be provided to you free of charge.

With a little dedication and some conscientious time and effort, you will discover the right medical health information to meet your needs.

This is your life. Go for it.

Good luck and good searching!

Paul J. Krupin
Kennewick, Washington

Summary of the Best Health Magic Search Words

Learn about Search Engines

Search engines

Search engine watch

Search engine showdown

Search engine comparison chart

invisible Web

invisible Web tutorial

The Minus Dot Com Trick

~.com.

<Subject> <topic> ...-.com...

-.com .org

<Subject> <topic> ...-.com .org

Learning Words & Internet Words

<Disease Words> <Learning Words> <Internet Words>

<Disease Words> <Skill word> tutorial

<Disease Words> online database

<Disease Words> online directory

<Source Word> searchable database

The Add a Word Technique

<Word # 1> <Word # 2> <Word # 3> <Word # 4>

Search String Word Groups

<Disease Words>

<Medical Specialty Words>

<Anatomy Words>

<Medical Action Words>

<Medical Issue Words>

<Symptom Words>

<Learning Words>

<Internet Words>

<Source Words>

<Location Words>

<Time Words>

The Search String Technique

<Word Group 1> <Word Group 2> <Word Group 3>

<Disease Word> <Medical Action Word> <Symptom Word>

Search Word Rotation

<Disease Word> <Medical Action Word #1> <Symptom Word>
<Disease Word> <Medical Action Word #2> <Symptom Word>
<Disease Word> <Medical Action Word #3> <Symptom Word>
<Disease Word> <Medical Action Word> <Symptom Word #1>
<Disease Word> <Medical Action Word> <Symptom Word #2>
<Disease Word> <Medical Action Word> <Symptom Word #3>

Concept or Phrase Searching and Exact Quote Searching

How to deal with <Disease Word>
Managing Your <Medical Issue Word>
Questions to Ask Your Doctor <Disease Word>

Information in Different Languages/From Specific Countries

<Disease Word> <Learning Words> <Internet Words> <Language Word> <Location Words>
<Disease Word> <Learning Words> <Internet Words> <Country Code>

Searching to Improve General Knowledge

<Disease Word> <Learning Words>
<Disease Word> <Learning Words> <Internet Words>

Searching to Improve Skills

<Medical Issue Word> <Medical Action Word> <Learning Words> <Internet Words>
<Medical Issue Word> <Medical Action Word> <Symptom Words> <Learning Words> <Internet Words>

Searching for Specific Facility Services or Providers

<Medical Issue Word> <Medical Action Word> <Learning Words> <Internet Words>
<Medical Issue Word> <Medical Specialty Words> <Learning Words> <Internet Words>
<Medical Issue Word> <Medical Action Word> <Facility Words> <Source Words> <Location Words>
<Disease Words> <Source Words> online directory
<Disease Words> <Source Words> online database
<Disease Words> <Business Words> <Learning Words> <Internet Words> <Source Words>
<Disease Words> <Government Words> <Learning Words> <Internet Words> <Source Words>
<Disease Words> <Association Words> <Learning Words> <Internet Words> <Source Words>
<Disease Words> <Organization Words> <Learning Words> <Internet Words>
<Disease Words> <Community Words> <Learning Words> <Internet Words>
<Disease Words> <Media Words> <Learning Words> <Internet Words> <Source Words>

Searching to Meet Specific Personal Needs or Desires

<Medical Issue Word> <Medical Action Word> <Source Words> <Location Words> <Date Words>
<Medical Issue Word> <Medical Action Word> <Facility Words> <Source Words> <Location Words>
<Medical Issue Word> <Medical Specialty Words> <Source Words> <Location Words>

Index

3w Virtual Library, the, 10

About.com, 10

abuse, 52, 57, 62, 66, 88, 96, 98–99, 109, 111, 123, 126, 134, 137

add a word, 16, 18, 22, 24–25, 30–31, 141

advanced searches, 16

age words, 24–25, 27–28, 40, 51, 87, 108

age, gender, family & culture words, 40, 51, 104

aging, elder care, long–term care, 62–63

all about search engines, 7, 9, 11, 13, 40

all the web, 7, 9, 11

allergies, asthma, & immunology, 62, 64

Alta Vista, 9, 17

alternative health & medical treatment, 62, 65–66

anatomy words, 24, 40, 43–44, 54–55, 67, 69, 72, 75, 77–78, 80, 85, 90, 94, 97, 100, 105–106, 110, 116, 141

Ask Jeeves, 11

association words, 24, 129–130, 142

associations, 12, 29–30, 41, 58, 72, 95, 102, 112, 123, 128–131, 148

automatic plurals, 17

avoiding disaster, 137

body part words, 24, 40, 44–45, 47, 55, 113

bones, muscles, joints, 62, 68, 70

boolean terms, 16

Britannica, 10

business words, 142

cancer care & treatment, 62, 70–71

case sensitivity, 17

CBI, 120–122

cellular biology, 40, 45, 126

CERN, 10

chiropractic care, 62, 72

Chubba, 11

city, 28–30, 83, 111, 127–129, 131, 147, 151

colds and the flu, 62, 73

colleges, 30, 41, 58, 131–132

community organizations, 30, 41

companies & corporations, 29, 41, 58, 123, 128

companies by name, 29

companies, 3, 12–13, 19, 29–30, 41, 58, 95, 107, 120, 123, 128–129, 148

complex medical health search strings, 55

concept searching, 18, 31, 142

conclusion, 137, 139

corporations, 29, 41, 58, 123, 128

country or culture words, 24

creating search strings, 5, 22, 55, 150

critical business information, 120–121

culture words, 24, 40, 51–52, 55, 104

Cyber 411, 11

database, 8, 16, 20–22, 30–31,
    42–43, 46, 83, 85, 94–98, 110,
    114, 118, 124, 126, 128, 130,
    133, 141–142, 148
death & dying, 62, 74–75
default settings:, 17
desktop search utilities, 13
detailed phrase searching, 33
diabetes, hormonal & immune
    system, 62, 77
digestive system & gastrointestinal
    illness, 62, 78
disease words, 24–25, 31, 40, 42–43,
    46–48, 54–56, 58–59, 64–65,
    67, 69, 71–73, 76–78, 80–81,
    86–87, 91, 93–94, 97–101,
    105, 107–108, 116–117, 130,
    141–142
doctor & medical specialty words,
    49, 89, 142
doctors & health care professionals,
    123
Dogpile, 11
ears and hearing, 62, 80
eating & nutrition, 62, 79, 81, 114
educational institutions, 30, 58, 123,
    131
emergency care, 77, 125
ethnic, 52–53, 104
Evans, Meryl K., xi–xii
exact quote searching, 33–34, 142
Excite, 9, 17
eye care & vision, 62, 85, 88
family relation words, 52
family words, 24, 40, 51–52, 64,
    73–74, 87, 98
federal government agencies, 19, 29
field searching, 17
foot care, 62, 77, 89
fraternal organizations, 30, 130
fraud, 123–124, 126, 134, 137–138

free stuff, 20, 123, 135
gender words, 24, 28, 40, 51–52, 108
getting started, 3–4
going from ideas to action, 120
Google, 5, 8–9, 17–18, 23, 34–35,
    103
government agencies, 3, 10, 12,
    19–20, 23, 29, 34, 58, 123,
    127–128, 138, 148
government words, 40, 74, 127–128,
    142
government, 3, 10, 12, 18–20, 23,
    29–30, 34, 40, 54, 58, 64, 74,
    102, 106, 121, 123, 126–128,
    130, 133, 138, 142, 147–148
headache and migraine, 62, 92
heart disease and cardiology, 62, 90
hospitals and health care facilities,
    123–124
Hotbot, 8–9
how to use this book, 4
human anatomy words, 40, 43–44
immune system disorders, 62, 77
improve your general knowledge,
    58–59
index, 7–9, 20, 42–44, 50, 68, 78, 85,
    91, 96, 110, 114, 126–127,
    132, 143, 145
industry words, 24, 133
infections, 56, 62, 69, 76, 79, 82,
    87–88, 93–94, 96, 107, 117
Inference Fund, 11
institutions, 10, 29–30, 58–59, 119,
    122–123, 129, 131, 134
Internet words, 3, 12, 21, 24–25, 30,
    35, 38, 40, 46, 54–55, 61, 114,
    122, 127–129, 131–133,
    141–142
invisible web, the, 11–12, 19, 141
Iwon, 9
kids search engines, 13

language, 35, 40, 75, 142
learning words, 12, 19–20, 24–25,
    30, 38, 40, 42, 46, 54–55, 61,
    63–64, 67–68, 70, 72–75,
    77–78, 80–81, 83, 85, 87, 89,
    91–95, 97–98, 100, 102–103,
    105–106, 108, 112, 114, 116,
    118, 127–129, 131–133,
    141–142
legal questions, 123, 134
Library of Congress, 10
location words, 24, 58–59, 97, 102,
    108, 112, 141–142
Looksmart, 10
lung diseases, 73, 94–95, 112
Lycos, 9, 17
Magellan, 9–10
MagicSearchWords.com, 5, 149–151
major search engines, 12–13, 17
Mamma, 11
media words, 24, 30, 72, 132, 142
medical action words, 24, 26–27,
    40, 48, 55–57, 64–65, 67, 69,
    71–73, 75–77, 79–80, 83, 86,
    90–92, 94–95, 98–99, 101,
    103–104, 106–110, 113, 117,
    141–142
medical education, 43, 92, 102, 123,
    126
medical scams, 134, 137–138
medical specialty words, 24, 40,
    49–51, 55, 89, 141–142
medication & drugs, 62, 93, 95–97,
    99, 108
men's health, 23, 62, 97–98, 134
mental health & psychiatry, 62, 98,
    105, 109
Meriam–Webster's dictionary, 19
meta–search engines, 11
Metacrawler, 11
metacrawlers, 13

Metafind, 11
Microsoft Internet Explorer, 4
minus dot com trick, the, 18–19, 49,
    58, 141
Mozilla, 4
Multi–search engines, 11
nervous system & neurology, 62,
    100
Netscape Navigator, 4
Netscape, 4, 10
news search engines, 13
nonprofit organizations, 30, 41, 58,
    130
One2seek, 11
Open Directory, 10
Opera, 4
operators, 16
organ system words, 45
organizations, 3, 12, 18–19, 23,
    29–31, 34, 41, 58, 72,
    119–120, 123, 125, 129–130
overview, 1, 39
paid listings search engines, 13
parting words, 138
philanthropic foundations, 30
phrase searching, 17–18, 31, 33, 142
physical & developmental
    disabilities, 62, 102
plastic surgery, 62, 102, 107, 112
professional and trade associations,
    29, 130
professional associations, 12, 29, 41,
    58, 72, 123, 129–130, 148
proximity searching, 17
purpose, 2, 24, 120, 137
rehabilitation, 26, 29, 48–49, 51, 55,
    57, 62–64, 71, 75, 102–103,
    110, 125
reward search engines, 13
robot, 8
scams, 134, 137–138

schools, 20, 30, 34, 41, 95, 123,
      131–132
search engine comparison chart, 12,
      141
search engine resources, 12
search engine showdown, 12, 141
search engine watch, 12, 141
search string technique, the, 3, 15,
      18, 24, 141
search string word groups, 23–24,
      29, 33, 40–42, 53–55, 61, 141
search strings, 2–3, 5, 10, 12, 16,
      20–22, 27, 29, 35, 38, 41–42,
      44, 49, 51, 53–55, 61, 119,
      132, 135, 138, 150
search tool, 8
search word rotation, 2, 26, 38, 56,
      141–142
selecting the magic search words,
      23, 53
sex & fertility, 62, 103–104, 117
simple medical health search
      strings, 55
simple phrase searching, 31
simple searches, 15, 23
skin care, 62, 106–107, 117
sleep disorders, 62, 99, 108
social problems, physical, sexual
      problems, 62, 109
software, 4, 7, 11–13, 128
source words, 24, 29, 38, 57–59,
      119, 141–142
spaces, 17
special tactics for creating search
      strings, 22

special topics in medical health
      care, 122
specialized search databases, 11, 13,
      132
specialty search engines, 13
specific goals for searching, 41
spider, 8, 13
stop words, 17, 34
substance abuse, 62, 98, 109, 111
surgery, 49, 62, 71, 85, 90–91,
      101–102, 107, 111–113,
      116–117, 124–125
symptom words, 24, 40, 47, 54–55,
      63, 65, 68–70, 73, 79–80, 82,
      86, 92, 95, 100, 105, 107, 110,
      117, 141–142
synonyms, 23–24, 27, 38, 46
tests, tools and calculators, 62, 113
thesaurus, 24
time words, 4, 24, 42, 56–57, 59, 141
trade groups, 30, 130
travel and health, 62, 115
true search engines, 7–9
tutorial, 12, 19–21, 44–45, 116, 135,
      141, 148
universities, 3, 10, 20, 30, 34, 41, 58,
      131–132
virtual libraries, 10–11
web directories, 9, 132
Webcrawler, 9
wild card truncations, 17
women's health, 23, 31, 62, 116
Yahoo, 10

Who is Paul J. Krupin?

Paul J. Krupin is a scientist and "once-upon-a-time" attorney. He has over 28 years of diverse professional government and industry experience in a variety of technology and project management disciplines at complex industrial, nuclear, waste management facilities. He has been employed with the State of Oregon, U.S. Department of Interior, U.S. Department of Agriculture, U.S. Department of Energy, several law firms, and private industry. He was an emergency medical technician (EMT) and a County Civil Defense Director in Idaho. Paul has spent a lifetime dedicated to helping the government, business, industry, small business and individuals come up with creative systems and innovative solutions to complex policy, legal, regulatory, and technological problems and challenges. He has worked on solving or contributing to the solutions of some of the world's worst pollution problems. His adventurous career in government infected him with a love of public service.

Born in New York City, he was raised in Franklin Square on Long Island. He received a Bachelors Degree from the University of Colorado in Boulder, Colorado, a Masters Degree from Oregon State University in Corvallis, Oregon, and a Juris Doctor with a special certificate in Dispute Resolution from Willamette University in Salem, Oregon.

In 1992, after vowing to never step into a courtroom again, Paul devoted his newly found spare time to becoming an author, publisher, Internet innovator, and professional problem solver. He has come up with numerous highly innovative Internet systems and solutions. He loves to identify and develop what he calls "technological force multipliers", which in his own words are, "success pathways en masse, made easy to use with technology."

He is a prolific writer whose pre-Internet creations included the Toll Free Environmental Directory which taught people how to search for environmental jobs and information long distance for free using toll-free numbers. He also wrote several fishing, hunting and archery books. He created several very popular highly specialized databases for government contractors including the National 8 A Minority and Economically Disadvantaged Company Directory & Databases series, Fed-Pro: The Federal Procurement Database, and DOD-Pro: The Department of Defense Procurement Database.

He discovered the Internet in 1994 and created a widely known media e-mail database called The US All Media E-Mail Directory. In 1996, he co-created, with Don Short of One World Telecommunications, IMEDIAFAX The Internet to Media Fax Service (www.Imediafax.com), an online service that allowed people to create their own custom targeted media lists and transmit news releases to them via fax and e-mail. Through IMEDIAFAX he has sent out millions of news releases each year. His clients include world-class companies, government agencies, professional associations and best selling authors on everything from *Chicken Soup for the Soul* to publicizing Internet and industry events to hard news journalists to syndicated columnists to electronic newsletters. Krupin's work is highly regarded in the publishing industry for his innovative Internet expertise and publicity achievements. He has touched the hearts and minds of millions of people.

The success stories and tactics of this remarkably successful Internet publicity service is chronicled in the highly rated book *Trash Proof News Releases*. He has developed sure-fire, proven strategies for getting publicity. His book covers the entire gamut of the how, why, when and where of news release construction, delivery and follow-up in today's fast evolving media environment. His book tantalizes you with real life PR success stories and proven tactics. His methods and services have helped hundreds of authors reach out to millions of people again and again.

Another of his Internet inventions is called www.EMailtotheMax.com, a free online tutorial which teaches business people how to avoid email liability and improve their Internet and email skills, productivity and capability in what he calls "Business Quality Email." For creating this remarkable free service, he was featured on CNN Financial.

The *Magic Search Words* series evolved out of a problem he identified in 1999. No one knew how to use search engines. He set to work and created a new concept that helps people learn how to identify and select the best words to enter in search engines to get the best information quicker and easier than ever before. The original book, called *Finding the Gold Online,* covered everything from kids' homework to teen competitions, scholarships, jobs, personal finance, business finance, and venture capital, all the way to retirement money. Mainstream east coast publishers rejected this book as all too encompassing and suggested that single topic books be created. Hence, the *Magic Search Words* Series with individual books dedicated to single topics was developed.

Paul derives his greatest personal satisfaction by touching and improving the lives of people. His goal is to help millions of people by giving them quicker and easier access to the best information on the Internet. With the creation of the Magic Search Word series, Paul is embarking on a global campaign to teach people how to get better information off the Internet than ever before. He feels most people believe that helping themselves using the Internet is more than just for fun, a job, or a career, it is a now a core value. Like the library was for our parents, the Internet has now become and will remain an intrinsic part of our lives and a significant factor that will affect the future of all humanity. He is a man with a vision, a heart, and a soaring spirit that is an inspiration to all who seek to improve themselves and the world around them.

To contact Paul for further information or to schedule him for a speech, training seminar, or workshop, please contact:

Direct Contact
P. O. Box 6726
Kennewick WA 99336
Tel: 509-545-2707 or 1-800-457-8746
Fax: 509-582-9865
To send e-mail write to info@MagicSearchWords.com
Visit www.MagicSearchWords.com

The Magic Search Word Series

Scholarships
Jobs
Health
Homework
Business
Law
Personal Finance
Animal and Pet Care
Environment

Free! Access to www.MagicSearchWords.com

Each of the Magic Search Words books provides you with free access to the custom programmed Magic Search Words web site.

MagicSearchWords.com automates the creation of search strings, so that creating search strings and submitting them to the best search engines is even faster and easier than ever.

You may go to www.MagicSearchWords.com anytime once you have purchased or downloaded a book.

Thank you for your interest in improving your life!

Get in Direct Contact—Quick Order Form

Fax Orders: 509-582-9865. Send this form.

Telephone Orders: Call 1-800-457-8746 toll free.
Or 509-545-2707. Have your credit card ready.

Email Orders: orders@MagicSearchWords.com

E-Books: Visit MagicSearchWords.com
WWW.MagicSearchWords.com

Internet: Visit MagicSearchWords.com
WWW.MagicSearchWords.com

Postal Orders: Direct Contact Publishing, Paul Krupin, PO Box 6726,
Kennewick WA 99336 USA, Tel: 509-545-2707

Please send the following books or products. I understand that I may return any of them for a full refund—for any reason, no questions asked.

_____ Quantity _____

_____ Quantity _____

_____ Quantity _____

_____ Quantity _____

Please send more FREE information on:

❑ Quantity/Premium Orders
❑ Other Books
❑ Speaking/Seminars/Workshops
❑ Mailing Lists
❑ Consulting
❑ Fund Raising

❑ Custom Programmed Magic Search Pages
❑ E-Mail & Web Based Training Courses
❑ News Releases & Media Kits
❑ The Magic Search Word Column
❑ Getting Publicity with IMEDIAFAX— The Internet To Media Fax Service

Name: _____

Address: _____

City: _____ State: _____ Zip: _____

E-Mail Address: _____

Sales Tax: Please add 8.5% for products shipped to Washington State addresses.

Shipping by US Priority Mail: U.S. $5.00 for first book and $2.00 for each additional book or product. International: $10.00 for first book and $5.00 for each additional book or product.

Payment: ❑ Cheque ❑ Credit Card — ❑ Visa ❑ MasterCard ❑ AMEX

Card Number: _____

Name on Card: _____

Exp. Date: _____

Address of Cardholder: _____